Praise for *Bod4God*

"In *Bod4God*, Steve Reynolds launches a full-scale frontal assault in the ongoing American war with obesity. His weapons—solid biblical teaching and modern fitness principles—serve more effectively than any smart bomb or stealth warplane in this battle. Reynolds's easy-to-understand, motivating plan can help even the most sedentary couch potato and is especially effective because it uses eternal wisdom from God's Word. Read *Bod4God* today and enlist in the healthy army of the fit and faithful!"

Darren Baroni, MD,
member, American College of Gastroenterology;
attending gastroenterologist

"Americans are in a fight for their health against a formidable 'Goliath': obesity. For years, the scientific community has told us what 'stones' will weaken the giant: good nutrition and exercise. But translating bench-top research to everyday living is the challenge. In *Bod4God*, Pastor Reynolds teaches us to be the 'David.' Armed with the slingshot of God's Word, you will launch healthy, up-to-date, scientific principles of exercise and nutrition to fight head-on the epidemic of obesity and topple the giant!"

Elizabeth P. Berbano, MD, MPH,
fellow, American College of Physicians;
certified, American Board of Internal Medicine

"It's been a blessing to partner with Pastor Reynolds and his congregation to provide Body & Soul as a key exercise strategy for the Bod4God program. In *Bod4God* there is a place for everyone to be successful. People of all ages and fitness levels have participated and seen improvements in cardiovascular fitness, strength, and flexibility. You will be encouraged and empowered by this book as you seek to improve your health and live a life of energy and vitality to God's glory."

Jeannie Blocher,
president, Body & Soul Fitness Ministries;
certified faculty, American Council on Exercise;
group fitness specialist, The Cooper Institute, Dallas, Texas

"One area of teaching that seems to be neglected in the church today is the area of our own health. The Bible tells us our bodies are the temple of the Holy Spirit, but do we really treat our bodies with that value in mind? That's why I'm so excited about *Bod4God*. Steve brings biblical principles to bear to help everyone with weight loss, exercise, and staying healthy. Every Christian should read this book—now!"

Jonathan Falwell,
pastor, Thomas Road Baptist Church, Lynchburg, Virginia

"*Bod4God* has produced more sustainable weight loss for its participants than any other program that I have been involved with in my twenty years as a dietitian. The focus on God and on losing weight for the right reasons was genuinely inspiring. The bonding, trust, and support of other participants helped keep the momentum going to achieve truly impressive results. Pastor Steve Reynolds is a great living example of God's power to transform."

Vivian Hutson,
registered dietician

"I have seen patients turn life-threatening conditions into manageable ones or even experience full restoration through lifestyle change, including diet and exercise. Pastor Reynolds shows the powerful effects of faith and lifestyle change in his transformation from an obese man to a man unburdened by weight and illness."

Ulrich Prinz, MD,
board-certified internist

"*Bod4God* is a much-needed reminder that God created our bodies as tools for His work and, as such, His Word has plenty to say about how we treat them. I first met Steve when he joined my coaching network, and I have been impressed with his insights. We would all be wise to take his words to heart. After all, our bodies are the handiwork of God, meant to aid us in carrying His message to the world. Without health, none of us can be very effective. Kudos to Steve for bringing this issue out of the dark!"

Nelson Searcy,
lead pastor, Journey Church;
founder, www.ChurchLeaderInsights.com

"Pastor Reynolds is a modern day prophet who strikes at the heart of the unhealthy lifestyle of most Americans and many members of the Christian community. His biblically based *Bod4God* is a credible program that could spark a movement toward weight control and healthier living. I heartily endorse this well-written, exciting book."

James M. Stern, MD,
fellow, American College of Surgeons

"Steve Reynolds has a great spirit of discipline and commitment to Jesus Christ, which is reflected in this book. For those who want to lose weight, you should read *Bod4God* to catch the *spirit*—not just the practical lessons but the spiritual lessons as well. Steve has put the right priority in weight loss—a person's relationship to God—and from that discipline concerning the 'temple of the Holy Spirit' they can lose weight."

Elmer L. Towns,
cofounder, Liberty University;
author, *Fasting for Spiritual Breakthrough*

BOD
4GOD

Also by Steve Reynolds

*Get Off the Couch: 6 Motivators to Help You
Lose Weight and Start Living*

Bod4God: The Four Keys to Weight Loss DVD Series

BOD 4 GOD

Twelve Weeks to Lasting Weight Loss

STEVE REYNOLDS

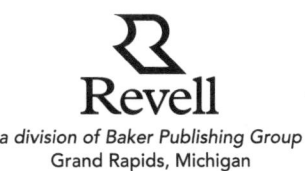

Revell

a division of Baker Publishing Group
Grand Rapids, Michigan

Published by Revell
a division of Baker Publishing Group
P.O. Box 6287, Grand Rapids, MI 49516-6287
www.revellbooks.com

Repackaged edition published 2016 by Revell

Previously published by Regal Books

Printed in the United States of America

Library of Congress Cataloging-in-Publication Data
Names: Reynolds, Steve (Pastor), author.
Title: Bod4God : twelve weeks to lasting weight loss / Steve Reynolds.
Other titles: Bod 4 God | Bod four God
Description: Grand Rapids : Revell, 2016. | Rev. ed. of: Bod4God : the four keys to weight loss.
   2009. | Includes bibliographical references.
Identifiers: LCCN 2016017404 | ISBN 9780800726812 (cloth)
Subjects: LCSH: Weight loss. | Weight loss—Religious aspects—Christianity. | Health—
   Religious aspects—Christianity. | Reducing diets.
Classification: LCC RM222.2 .R465 2016 | DDC 613.2/5—dc23
LC record available at https://lccn.loc.gov/2016017404

This publication is intended to provide helpful and informative material on the subjects addressed. Readers should consult their personal health professionals before adopting any of the suggestions in this book or drawing inferences from it. The author and publisher expressly disclaim responsibility for any adverse effects arising from the use or application of the information contained in this book.

In keeping with biblical principles of creation stewardship, Baker Publishing Group advocates the responsible use of our natural resources. As a member of the Green Press Initiative, our company uses recycled paper when possible. The text paper of this book is composed in part of post-consumer waste.

17   18   19   20   21   22   23   8   7   6   5   4   3   2

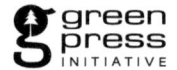

First, I dedicate this book to my God, who is the source of my life. I will spend the rest of my days on this earth honoring You with my body.

> According to my earnest expectation and hope that in nothing I shall be ashamed, but with all boldness, as always, so now also Christ will be magnified in my body, whether by life or by death.
>
> Philippians 1:20

Second, I dedicate this book to Debbie, my wife, who is my partner in life. I will spend the rest of my days on this earth loving you with my body.

> Who can find a virtuous wife?
> For her worth is far above rubies.
> The heart of her husband safely trusts her;
> So he will have no lack of gain.
> She does him good and not evil
> All the days of her life. . . .
> Her husband is known in the gates,
> When he sits among the elders of the land.
> Proverbs 31:10–12, 23

Third, I dedicate this book to Crystal, Sarah, and Jeremiah, my children, and their families, who are the inspiration for my life. I will spend the rest of my days influencing you with my body.

> I have no greater joy than to hear that my children walk in truth.
>
> 3 John 1:4

Contents

Acknowledgments

This was a team project.

I greatly appreciate the group of people who helped me develop this book, including:

My parents, for always supporting me. I love you both very much.

My family, for being my inspiration for living healthy and sacrificing time without me while I worked on this book.

My church family, members and staff of Capital Baptist Church in Annandale, Virginia, for your loyal support. It is truly an honor to serve as your pastor.

My colaborers, the leaders and participants in the Losing To Live Weight Loss Competitions throughout the country and the world. Your partnership is invaluable in the ongoing success of this movement.

My writing assistants, Jana Moritz and Gwen Ellis—thank you for all you did to help this busy pastor.

My mentors, the late Jerry Falwell and Elmer Towns, for your impact on my life and ministry.

My friend Carole Lewis, First Place 4 Health National Director Emeritus, for assistance in advancing this book. You are probably responsible for more weight loss among Christians than anyone in the history of the church.

My friends Gary Moritz and Pete Frenquelle for your creative contribution to this project.

My photographer, Randy Ritter, who took most of the pictures in this book.

My publisher, Baker Publishing Group, and especially Vicki Crumpton, for your guidance in producing a quality book.

My media contacts—thank you for helping to spread the Bod4God message around the country and the world.

My readers—you honor me for taking time out of your busy lives to read this book.

Foreword

I first met Pastor Steve Reynolds when he invited me to speak at one of his Losing To Live orientations. I was thrilled to be a part of this exciting ministry that had been gaining much publicity throughout the United States. Since that time Pastor Steve and I have partnered closely in promoting wellness and fighting obesity. He and I have the same passion for a healthy church community. He includes First Place 4 Health in his church wellness program. He also regularly speaks at our First Place 4 Health events and contributes to our monthly newsletter.

There are many things I admire about Steve Reynolds, but number one on the list is that he is a pastor who has lost over 130 pounds after struggling with his weight for many years and has beat the odds by keeping it off. He adopted a Bod4God lifestyle and was healed of high blood pressure, high cholesterol, and diabetes. Steve Reynolds is leading the wellness fight from a position of strength and vitality. He is rock solid.

Pastor Steve tells that his weighing more than 340 pounds was never challenged in his church because being overweight is acceptable in the Christian community today. However, after God showed him through the Bible how to lose weight and keep it off, he was willing to be the change agent starting in his church, and now thousands of people have literally lost tons of weight through his influence. He communicates an honest, biblical message of how to get and stay healthy.

In this book, *Bod4God: Twelve Weeks to Lasting Weight Loss*, you will learn four keys to lasting weight loss. These keys are enhanced by the spiritual component of faith in God, which sets this book apart. These wellness keys are practical, purposeful, powerful, and based on the Bible. These keys will unlock a new and healthy life for you. I have personally seen many lives radically changed by them. Steve Reynolds has compassion and concern for people who are in poor health and unable to effectively serve God because of their excess weight and sedentary lifestyle. He personally knows what it is like to experience extreme obesity and major weight loss, and now he has written this book for the individual who is finally willing to take what he calls "small steps to life."

As you run your race, I want you to run healthy, run steady, run with someone by your side, and run focused. Pastor Steve has done it, others are doing it, and you can do it. Whatever you do, keep your eyes on the prize and run strong. Whenever I feel like quitting, I go back to Hebrews 12:1–3, which has served as my flagship of hope and my wellness theology.

> Therefore we also, since we are surrounded by so great a cloud of witnesses, let us lay aside every weight, and the sin which so easily ensnares us, and let us run with endurance the race that is set before us, looking unto Jesus, the author and finisher of our faith, who for the joy that was set before Him endured the cross, despising the shame, and has sat down at the right hand of the throne of God. For consider Him who endured such hostility from sinners against Himself, lest you become weary and discouraged in your souls.

Through these three verses, and personal examples in people like Steve Reynolds, God has taught me to not give up. You may have a lot to overcome, just like Steve and I did. Being successful at anything in life requires discipline and sacrifice. It is no different when it comes to your health. Living a healthy life requires that you discipline and sacrifice yourself to not eat the things that are not good for you and to make the time to exercise and move your body. Unfortunately, words like *discipline* and *sacrifice* are countercultural today. Successful people overcome, learn from the past, and preserve their future legacy. What will your legacy be? This journey will not be easy. You will face obstacles, but you can overcome them. *Bod4God: Twelve Weeks to Lasting Weight Loss* will help you stay on track, and after twelve weeks, you will have a working knowledge of how to win at weight loss and how to sustain it.

This book is what the relevant church needs and is looking for—solid biblical keys of wellness. I am standing with Pastor Steve Reynolds in the fight against obesity. Obesity is no respecter of persons. It affects men, women, teens, children, pastors, and parishioners. When you consider the severe risks of obesity, I want to challenge you to run the race with us, read and apply this book, make weight loss a top priority, and begin to change like thousands of others have done. Be part of something bigger than yourself and fight with us. Don't let past fitness failures keep you from a balanced, healthy life. Start now and pursue your Bod4God, one day at a time and one pound at a time!

Vicki Heath
national director, First Place 4 Health;
author, *Don't Quit, Get Fit*

Before You Begin

A Word from Pastor Steve

You've picked up this book because you have a need to lose weight—or at least you have an interest in losing weight. Maybe you're tired of endless weight-loss plans and endless years of trying to get the numbers on that scale to start moving downward. Maybe you are feeling as if this is your last attempt to find something that will work. You've come to the right place. I can help you.

I understand what you've been through, because I've been through it too. I understand how frustrated you've become, because I've been frustrated too. Perhaps, like me, you've heard frightening news from your doctor, who has warned you to lose weight—now!

First of all, I want you to know that not only do I understand your situation, but I also care about it. I care about you. I've become so passionate about turning overweight people into losers that much of my life today is wrapped up in finding ways to help people change. I was a fat little kid who grew up, played football through college, vowed never to exercise again after I quit playing football, kept the promise, and ballooned to a weight of over 340 pounds. I heard my own doctor say those fearful words, "You have high blood pressure, high cholesterol, and diabetes." Even then, it took me a while to begin doing something about my obesity.

Then, with God's help, I found a way to begin taking small steps, and those small steps led to a new lifestyle. They led to life. That's what this book is all about—a path to a new life. I want to share what I've learned, because it works. I've lost more than 130 pounds and am still losing. I no longer need medications for high blood pressure, high cholesterol, and diabetes. Now I really feel good and have lots of energy. I'll share my secrets with you—all of them. You won't find them very profound or complicated, but I can promise you that if you start taking what I call "small steps to life," and you stick with them, they will work for you as they have for thousands of others, and they will lead to lasting weight loss.

What Is "Losing To Live"?

Christians are the most overweight people group in America. Losing To Live has been designed to confront and solve this problem. There are two ways to approach weight loss using this program: as a personal challenge or as a group competition. Losing To Live will show you how to lose weight and keep it off through establishing a Bod4God lifestyle. There are four keys to weight loss. They are:

1. Dedication: Honoring God with Your Body
2. Inspiration: Motivating Yourself for Change
3. Eat and Exercise: Managing Your Habits
4. Team: Building Your Circle of Support

See, I told you these four keys are not very complex! But they work, and they have made lasting weight loss possible for thousands of people. They can do the same thing for you.

Three Reasons Losing To Live Will Work for You

There are three unique aspects of Losing To Live that make it so effective. They are:

1. It is *biblical*. You will learn how to apply the Bible to your life in the area of losing weight and improving your health.

2. It is *personal*. You will learn how to craft your own individual lifestyle plan.

3. It is *incremental*. You will learn how to choose "small steps to life" that will slowly but surely lead you to lasting life change.

This powerful combination is what will make this plan so successful for you.

What It Takes to Be a Big Loser

The Bod4God Victory Guide at the end of each chapter helps you take the information in this book and make it personal in your life. It includes the Bod4God weekly thought, memory verse, reflection/application questions, and the Small Steps to Life Record. The thorough completion of these things will equip you to practice the four keys to weight loss. Big losers make the Victory Guide a high priority! A Bod4God Close-Up and Small Steps to Life Ideas have been provided to help you complete the Victory Guide and craft

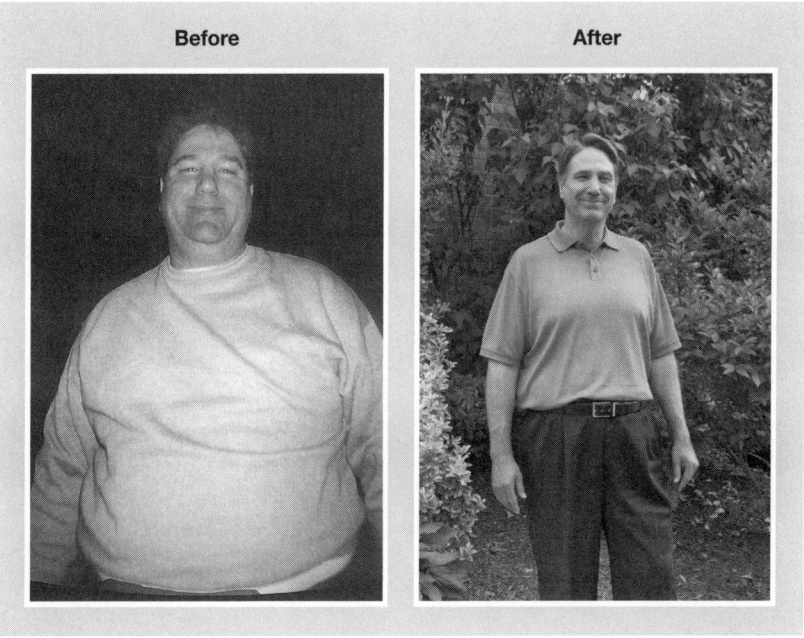

Before **After**

your new lifestyle plan along with a Victory Guide Chart on the following page to help you track your progress. The Bod4God Journal page allows you to make notes. Remember that *the victory is in the Victory Guide.*

So, are you ready for a weight-loss program that really works? Will you take the twelve weeks to lasting weight loss challenge? Then join the Losing To Live weight-loss program, and before you know it, you will have a Bod4God.

Celebrate and monitor your accomplishments as you complete the weekly Victory Guide assignments at the end of each chapter by putting a check mark in the designated box.

Victory Guide Chart

Week	Read *Bod4God* Chapter	Bod4God Thought	Memory Verse	Answer Questions	Do Small Steps to Life
1	The Anti-Fat Pastor		Colossians 1:16		
2	Losing to Live		Matthew 16:24–25		
3	*D* Is for Dedication		Galatians 5:16		
4	*D* Is for More Dedication		Romans 10:9		
5	*I* Is for Inspiration		John 10:10		
6	*I* Is for More Inspiration		Philippians 4:13		
7	*E* Is for Eat		1 Thessalonians 4:4		
8	*E* Is for Exercise		1 Corinthians 10:31		
9	*T* Is for Team: A Personal Challenge		Psalm 51:12		
10	*T* Is for Team: A Group Competition		Ecclesiastes 4:9		
11	Frequently Asked Questions		1 Peter 3:15		
12	Your Lifestyle Plan		Review		

My Progress Report

In order to know what progress you are making, you need a place to record where you began and whether you are losing or gaining weight. Please fill out the information requested below. Each week for twelve weeks, record your progress. It's important, so be faithful.

Name: .... Start Date: .... End Date: ....

My Starting Weight: .... My Final Weight: .... Goal: ....

	My Starting Measurements:		**My Ending Measurements:**
Neck:	....	Neck:	....
Arm (Bicep):	....	Arm (Bicep):	....
Chest:	....	Chest:	....
Waist:	....	Waist:	....
Hips:	....	Hips:	....
Thigh:	....	Thigh:	....
Calf:	....	Calf:	....

My Weight Loss

Week	+ / –	Week	+ / –
1		7	
2		8	
3		9	
4		10	
5		11	
6		12	

The Anti-Fat Pastor

Your Body Was Made by God and for God

For by Him all things were created that are in heaven and that are on earth, visible and invisible, whether thrones or dominions or principalities or powers. All things were created through Him and for Him.

Colossians 1:16

Calling the Flock to God, Away from the Fridge:
Northern Virginia Pastor Joins Ranks of Faithful Eyeing Scales
The Washington Post, Monday, January 22, 2007

There it was in bold print and on the front page of the *Washington Post*, and it was about me—me, Steve Reynolds, a local pastor who got sick and tired of being sick and tired and decided to do something about it, starting with losing weight. It's a long story. So let's rewind to the beginning, back to where weight began to be a problem for me.

I grew up in a Southern blue-collar family in a small town. My background was very simple. My parents didn't graduate from high school. No one in our family had ever graduated from college until my brother and I did. But here I was, pastor of a church in suburban Washington, DC, and dealing with my own weight problem, when all of a sudden I wound up on the front page of a major metropolitan newspaper, the *Washington Post*. I'm definitely not a front-page-of-the-paper kind of guy. First came the article and then came many interviews, including one with Neil Cavuto of Fox News. Neil was the first person to label me the "Anti-Fat Pastor."

I had struggled with weight all my life. In first grade, when most kids weigh about 45 pounds, I weighed more than a hundred—104 to be exact. My mother said that when I was a baby, I had a super-sensitive stomach. I had a tough time keeping food down, but Mom must have succeeded in getting some of the food to stay down because I began to pack on weight.

I'm proud of my Southern heritage, but you probably know about the traditional Southern diet. I ate a lot of fried chicken, pecan pie, sweet tea—lots of grease and sugar in my food. My diet was as unhealthy as it could be. It's not uncommon to see overweight kids today, but in 1963, it was rather unusual, and I looked unusual. I stood out in the class picture. Mom had to shop in the "husky boys" clothing section of the store. I wasn't just a little bit overweight; I had childhood obesity. By the time I started being concerned about my weight, I'd been overweight for many years.

Throughout much of my life, I thought I was just fine. I even poked fun at people who were lean and fit. I'd say things like, "Where's the beef, skinny guy? Real men eat red meat," and "Who, me? Eat salad? Salads are for sissies." Probably, if the truth were told, I was covering up a low self-image. Most overweight people do.

In grade school, I started playing sports. I was a big kid, and at that time, kids were ranked first by age and then by weight. The coaches would ask, "How old are you?" "Eight," I'd answer. Then, because my weight was far above the weight set for kids my age, and because I might hurt some of the smaller eight-year-olds when playing with them, I was bumped up to the next division. I had to play with older kids. There were times when I was bumped up two divisions. I never did play with kids my own age.

In some ways, being in a higher division worked to my advantage. I became a pretty good football player and got offers from half a dozen small colleges. I accepted one at Liberty University in Virginia. I was a four-year starter on Liberty's football team, and I was fortunate to go through college on a full football scholarship. I thank the Lord for that scholarship, but to keep and develop my football skills and my strength, I had to stay active throughout the year. College football was, and is, a year-round sport. That helped me maintain a good weight.

I started playing football when I was about eight years old, and I played all the way through until I was twenty-two. Then, when I finished, I made myself a promise. "Nobody's ever going to make me exercise again for the rest of my life." I was sick of everything associated with playing football—the push-ups, the running, the exhaustion, the pain, the pressure. I've broken plenty of promises in my life, but unfortunately, I kept this one.

When I graduated from college, I went on to seminary. I ate what I wanted to eat, and I kept my promise not to exercise. After seminary, I was ordained, and my beautiful bride, Debbie, and I were excited about our future together. We felt called to be church planters. In the fall of 1982, I launched a new church plant just outside Washington, DC. I soon learned that only one of ten new churches becomes successfully established; 90 percent fail. *Hmm.* I had just begun to work in a field with a 90 percent failure rate. I don't like to fail, and I wasn't about to fail at establishing this church. I was determined to work as hard as I could to make this church plant successful. I wanted my tombstone to read, "Here is a man who prayed like it all depended on God and worked like it all depended on him."

The good news is the church started to grow; the bad news is so did I. I worked as hard as I could during the day. I knocked on doors and contacted people about our new church. No one had asked me to come here and start a church, so I had to go out and let people know about it. When I came home late in the evening, I'd sit down in my La-Z-Boy recliner. (I've worn out three chairs so far in my life, and I plan to go to the grave still owning some kind of La-Z-Boy chair.) A real man has a La-Z-Boy chair, and when I'm in mine, I hold the remote. Anybody can sit in my chair and hold the remote when I'm not home, but when I come in, you need to get out of my chair and hand over the remote so nobody will get hurt. So as soon as I'd greeted my family, I'd get into my chair and start eating.

I've even thought about bringing my chair to church and doing a series on things I've learned sitting in my chair. One of the things I could teach is how to eat ice cream. Late at night, in that La-Z-Boy, I ate every kind of food in general, and ice cream in particular. I loved ice cream. I was truly *addicted* to it. I ate it every night. I had seen the ice cream eating pattern modeled every day of my childhood, and we are shaped by what we see modeled for us. To this day, my dad eats ice cream every night. I've seen him polish off a half gallon of ice cream at a time. Dad, however, is only a little overweight because he walks regularly. I, on the other hand, faithfully kept my promise never to exercise again.

I had worked at a grocery store for years, so when Debbie and I got married, I volunteered to do the grocery shopping for our family. I still shop for the family's groceries. When I went shopping for food, I'd search for ice cream that was on sale and then buy six half gallons at a time. As church planters, we were struggling financially, but I had to have my ice cream. I'd go down the aisle looking for whatever was on sale. When Breyer's chocolate chip was on sale, that was especially exciting. I didn't know if the kids were going to have Pampers, but no matter how tough times were, I was going to have my ice cream. Here I was, not exercising and eating whatever I wanted. I grew and grew and grew to 340 pounds. I had terrible health: high blood pressure, high cholesterol, and diabetes. I was literally digging my grave with a knife, fork, and, of course, an ice cream spoon.

Diabetes will kill you. The disease runs in my family, and while I hoped I'd never get it, I wasn't too surprised when I was diagnosed with it. I didn't ask what I could do to change the situation. I didn't even consider a lifestyle change. I just looked at the doctor and asked, "What pills do I need to take to control this?" He gave me prescriptions, and I began taking eight pills a day for the diabetes and other health-related problems.

This went on for six years. Then I heard that if you lose weight it might help to control diabetes. I learned that losing weight could also help control high blood pressure, high cholesterol, and a number of other illnesses, some of which I already had. Diabetes is not always a weight-related issue, and I wouldn't want anyone reading this book to start trying to lose weight and stop taking insulin. If you have diabetes, you need to work carefully with your medical doctor to monitor your condition.

Diabetes can also be hereditary. My grandfather was a skinny, muscular farmer who was probably never overweight a day in his life, *and* he was a diabetic. My mother is a diabetic who *is* overweight. Well, I had diabetes *and* I was definitely overweight. *Would I be able to control my diabetes if I lost weight?* I wondered.

I Changed My Habits and God Changed My Health

God had begun to work in my heart, and He was telling me I needed to do something about my overeating and lack of exercise. Slowly, I began the journey of trying to improve my health. At first, the issue was so personal that I told no one. I kept it between God and me. I knew I could never lose weight and be fit without God's intervention. I began to pray and seek His direction. I started losing weight, and when I had lost 70 pounds, my high blood pressure, high cholesterol, and diabetes were brought under control. To this day, I'm free from those illnesses.

God is faithful, and He is able. He led me to a passage in His Word that directly addressed the issues I was facing. It was the Colossians passage at the beginning of this chapter. I learned that everything that exists was created by Him and for Him. That includes me. If He was in control of all things, then He was in control of my life, and if I'd let Him, He could be in control of my weight issues too. It was a wonderful revelation!

As I prayed and meditated on this Scripture, God gave me a step-by-step prescription for making a huge change in my life—a change I'm going to share in the pages of this book. Once I began to follow it, I began to see results. Yes, I saw physical changes, but I also saw spiritual changes. My faith increased with each change I made and each pound I shed. I knew I'd discovered something important and it was my responsibility to share what I'd learned with my church and my community. I realized that Christians are the most overweight people group on earth.[1] We are more overweight than Muslims, Hindus, Buddhists, and every other religion you can name. (More about this later.)

Christians should be the healthiest people group, especially when we consider the physical condition of Jesus Christ, our founder and leader. Jesus's earthly father, Joseph, was likely a carpenter, and Jesus took up the trade. He would have had to lift heavy pieces of wood and would have had to saw them into boards by hand. What strength this would have required. After He began His public ministry, Jesus was always on the move. We know from Scripture, as referenced in Matthew 15:21–29, that Jesus walked from Sidon to Tyre, which would have been a forty-mile trip in one day. Jesus's whole life involved exercise, and He would have had to have been in great physical condition.

Little Christs

When God spoke to me about my weight, I finally faced my situation. I took the first step. I decided to go to the Bible for help. Philippians 1:20–21 says, "Christ will be magnified in my body, whether by life or by death. For to me, to live is Christ, and to die is gain." Christ wanted to be magnified in my body! That was amazing!

I'm a Christian, and "Christian" means "little Christ." In other words, we are to be Christlike. Our leader—Jesus Christ—was in such great physical condition that He could walk 40 miles, not in Reeboks but in leather sandals; and yet His followers on this planet are unhealthy, overweight, sedentary couch potatoes. That concerns me, and it ought to concern you. God wants to address this condition not only in our bodies but in our churches as well. God wants to help us in this area of weight management.

What the Bible Says

Colossians 1:16 says that "all things were created through Him and for Him." That means everything in heaven, everything on earth, everything visible, and everything invisible. He set up thrones, dominions, rulers, and authorities. Everything that exists has been created *by* Christ and *for* Him—even your body. God is your Creator. He has given you life. We Christians are strong on the Creator aspect of God's character, but we are weak in the area of a God who is also our Controller. He must also be the Controller of our lives. If we are made for God, then our bodies belong to God. And that's what this program is all about.

The word *body* is found 179 times in the Bible. I started studying those passages. Approximately one-third of them talk about our future bodies in heaven. They will be perfect and will not be affected by what we eat or don't eat—including ice cream. We will have heavenly bodies; but today, we are still living in earthly bodies. I started studying the remaining Scripture references to body. Out of my study, God showed me the four keys to lasting weight loss. As I mentioned, those keys are:

- Dedication: Honoring God with Your Body
- Inspiration: Motivating Yourself for Change

- Eat and Exercise: Managing Your Habits
- Team: Building Your Circle of Support

Then God helped me apply those keys and I started losing weight. People noticed and began to ask what plan I was on to lose weight. I had so many people ask me what I was doing that I decided to do a sermon series on getting a body for God. I called it "Bod4God."

I'm a Loser

Four times a year I send out a card listing my sermon series. One of those times in 2007, I put the Bod4God topic on the card. Thousands of people got the mailing, including a reporter from the *Washington Post*. She called me and said, "Pastor, I got the postcard and it sounds pretty interesting. A church talking about weight loss? That's a little unusual. I'd like to come hear those messages." Of course, I invited her to come. She came and wrote the article we talked about earlier. I expected it to appear on some back page of the *Washington Post*. However, there it was, right on the front page. The article was picked up by the Associated Press and literally went all over the world. I knew then that God was up to something. Then came the Fox News interview and a lot of others, and I became the "Anti-Fat Pastor."

Today, I am proud to announce that I'm a loser. I'm proud that I've lost more than 100 pounds. My diabetes is controlled by lifestyle. While I understand that not every diabetic can control the disease by losing weight, it has worked for me and I am thankful. I know that someday the diabetes might return since it is in my family genetics, but for now, I don't have it.

I would like nothing better than to see whole churches full of losers. My goal at my church—Capital Baptist Church—is to be the greatest losing church in America. We have lost over 12 tons so far! What about you? What about your church? I'm not here to judge anyone or any church about weight. I still need to lose more weight myself, and since I have struggled with weight all my life, I know the difficult part for me will be keeping the weight off. I'll struggle with it to the end of my days, but I am confident that by applying all that I present to you in this book, I can keep the weight off.

Small Steps to Life Will Work for You

Losing weight may seem impossible to you. Perhaps you've tried every diet plan known to man and none have worked. One of the main reasons those fad diets don't work is that they ask you to do too much too soon. When that happens, you get frustrated and quit. I understand, so I want to encourage you to start with small steps to life that you can do. If you do just a few steps in the areas of eating and exercising the first week, and then you are faithful to do those steps every day, the following week you will be able to add more steps that will help you gradually move toward weight-loss success. What you are building is a new lifestyle—one that will be filled with health and energy.

In this program, the difference between weight loss and no weight loss is based on what you do about creating small steps to life. People who consistently implement these small steps will lose weight; those who don't implement any small steps will not lose weight.

Pastor Steve's Small Steps to Life

To get started on my weight-loss and healthy body quest, I consistently took this small spiritual step to life:

> I had (and continue to have) a special time with God every day to fill up the inner man. He truly is my portion (see Psalm 119:57). When my inner man has been stuffed full, my physical man won't be so hungry, and I will have better control over what I eat.

Here are some of the food substitution small steps that worked for me:

- Instead of a bagel, I eat a protein health bar.
- Instead of ice cream, I eat Greek nonfat yogurt.
- Instead of diet sodas, I drink water during the day.
- I went from eating no fruit to eating an apple a day.
- I went from eating a hamburger and fries to eating chicken salad with a small amount of low-fat dressing.
- Instead of using mayonnaise on sandwiches, I use mustard.

- Instead of fried chips and dip, I eat baked chips and salsa.
- Instead of eating lots of beef, I eat lots of chicken and some fish.
- Instead of white bread, I eat whole-grain bread.
- Instead of fried foods, I eat baked foods (reduces the amount of fat).
- Instead of greasy French fries, I eat baked sweet potatoes.
- Instead of vegetable oil, I use olive oil (a monounsaturated oil—the good kind of fat!).
- Instead of high-fat creamer, I use fat-free creamer.
- I went from taking no vitamins to taking vitamins daily.
- I went from eating no kale to eating lots of kale (a dark green, highly nutritious vegetable).
- I went from eating no blueberries to eating lots of blueberries (a powerful antioxidant food).
- I stopped eating canned food (can contain lots of salt and preservatives) and began eating fresh or frozen food.
- I went from eating peanut butter and crackers to eating almonds (a good source of protein and monounsaturated fat).
- I went from using Sweet 'n' Low to using Stevia (a sweetener that has a negligible effect on blood glucose levels).
- I stopped eating mostly processed foods and began eating whole, unprocessed foods.
- I went from taking in no flaxseed to eating ground flaxseed on cereals, salads, in drinks, and so on (good for heart health and cholesterol levels).

To get started with exercise, I intentionally moved more. I would go out of my way to walk farther and put more effort in my daily activities. I then went to the gym and started walking on the treadmill and lifting weights. I started slowly and gradually increased my time on the treadmill and my weight-training repetitions.

Your Small Steps to Life

Now it's your turn to craft your own individual lifestyle plan. Throughout this book, you will find some ideas for small steps to life. These ideas may or may not work for you. You must research activities and ways to move that you will enjoy and discover healthy habits that you can do for the rest of your life. Start slowly and increase activity gradually, but above all, be consistent. Over a period of time, your small steps will take you a great distance and will help you achieve lasting weight loss. This is not just another diet plan that you do for a little while and then give up on. You are committing yourself to a lifestyle plan that will help you lose weight and keep it off.

Small Steps to Life Ideas

What Do You Need to Know about H$_2$O?

You must drink an adequate amount of water to be healthy and lose weight, so every week I am going to give you a little more information about water's importance. Every weight-loss program advocates drinking more water than most of us drink on a regular basis. Why? Many times we are not hungry but thirsty. Our brains interpret thirst as hunger, and we start grazing for something to satisfy the body's need. The Mayo Clinic website, on the subject of how much water to drink, says that we need to replace the fluids our bodies lose each day. The average output of urine is about 6.3 cups per day for an adult. In addition, other bodily processes such as breathing and sweating account for additional fluid loss. Fluid loss must be replaced on a daily basis.[2]

How much water should you drink? You need to take your weight in pounds, divide it in half, and then convert the number of pounds into ounces. So if you weigh 200 pounds, you should be drinking 100 ounces of water a day. Perhaps you are among those who say they don't like to drink water. That's because you have never tried it. Once you start drinking enough water, your body will crave it and will respond positively to being well hydrated.

There is a debate about whether other fluids such as soft drinks, fruit juice, and iced teas should be counted as water intake. While they are liquid, anything with caffeine in it acts as a diuretic and further strips water from your system. Fruit juices and tea with sugar—natural or added sugar—are processed by the body as food. The best solution is to drink plain water and drink enough so that you rarely feel thirsty and your urine is only slightly yellow.

Do this one small step of drinking more water each day, and stay with it. It *will* make a difference. Since our intent is to build a new lifestyle, drinking enough water is a good way to begin.[3]

Small Food Step

I began to get control of my eating by practicing portion-controlled eating. Remember, your stomach is about the size of your fist, so don't eat the size of your head. Your approach should be to slowly and systematically decrease the unhealthy things you are eating and slowly and systematically increase the good things you should be eating. This approach works because it allows you to retrain your taste buds and develop the right food cravings.

Small Exercise Step

Walk more. Park your car at the far perimeter of the shopping center and walk rather than parking close and moving your car every time you change stores. Although this is an incredibly small thing, it will get you started on a larger exercise program.

Bod4God Victory Guide

The Bod4God Victory Guide at the end of each chapter is the place where you will take the information in this book and make it personal in your life. It includes the Bod4God weekly thought, memory verse, reflection/application questions, and the Small Steps to Life Record. The thorough completion of these things will equip you to practice the four keys to weight loss. Big losers make the Victory Guide a high priority! Remember that *the victory is in the Victory Guide*. Each week record your progress on My Progress Report located on page 22.

Week 1: The Anti-Fat Pastor

Bod4God Thought

Your body was made by God and for God.

Bod4God Memory Verse

For by Him all things were created that are in heaven and that are on earth, visible and invisible, whether thrones or dominions or principalities or powers. All things were created through Him and for Him. (Colossians 1:16)

Bod4God Reflection/Application Questions

1. In Colossians 1:16, notice the two ways you were created: through God and for God. What does it mean to you to be created through God? What does it mean to you to be created for God?

....

....

....

....

....

2. In what ways do you think this verse is related to your struggle to get your weight under control and become healthier?

....

....

....

....

....

3. How much of a role, if any, has your childhood and social culture played in your struggle with weight?

....

....

....

....

....

4. In this chapter, I make a connection between the bad habits I learned from my family growing up and the behaviors I developed on my own. Note that I am careful not to place the blame on my family for the struggles I have had with my weight as an adult. Which of the following might you be tempted to blame for your struggle with weight?

...... Parents	...... Metabolism	...... Genetics
...... Stress	...... Heritage	...... Gender
...... God	...... Self	...... Stage of Life
...... Occupation	...... Environment	...... Finances
...... Other:		

5. Two of the habits that put me in the situation of being severely overweight included my nightly routines of La-Z-Boy lounging and eating ice cream. What are some habits that have negatively impacted your health?

....

....

....

....

....

6. Developing diabetes, along with my deep desire to live, was my motivation to lose weight and lead a healthier lifestyle. What is your motivation for physical change?

....

....

....

....

....

7. How would you assess your past attempts to lose weight and get healthy? What did you do to make your weight go up or down?

....

....

....

....

....

8. Think about the times when you lost or gained a major amount of weight. What was going on in your life at that time? School activities? Marriage? A new baby? A career or job change? The death of a friend, a family member, or a pet? Write down what you did in response to these events that caused your weight to go up or down.

....

....

....

....

....

Bod4God Small Steps to Life Record

What "Skinny Things" Will You Do This Week?

Fill out this chart each week by indicating: (1) what you will do to eat less to live; (2) what you will do to exercise more to live; and (3) how many average daily ounces of water you will drink. Pick only a few things, and stick with them. Remember that weight loss and maintenance require you to *eat less* and *exercise more*.

Sun.	
Mon.	
Tues.	
Wed.	
Thurs.	
Fri.	
Sat.	

My Bod4God Journal

Teach me, O LORD, the way of Your statutes, and I shall keep it to the end.

Psalm 119:33

Record what God is telling you to do this week to apply the four keys to lasting weight loss.

Dedication: Honoring God with My Body

....

....

....

....

Inspiration: Motivating Myself for Change

....

....

....

....

....

Eat and Exercise: Managing My Habits

....

....

....

....

....

Team: Building My Circle of Support

....

....

....

....

Losing To Live

Eat Less and Exercise More

Then Jesus said to His disciples, "If anyone desires to come after Me, let him deny himself, and take up his cross, and follow Me. For whoever desires to save his life will lose it, but whoever loses his life for My sake will find it."

Matthew 16:24–25

This passage reflects a major theme of Jesus's preaching. Everywhere He went, He wanted people to know, "Hey, you want life? Who doesn't? Here's how you get it. Deny yourself, take up your cross, and follow Me." God burned this passage into my heart. It has probably had more influence on my life than any other passage of Scripture. For me, incorporating this passage into my life became the challenge of losing weight so that I could live—I call it "losing to live."

God created our bodies, and He created them for Himself. Your body is the temple of the Holy Spirit. It is a holy place. You may ask, "Is God really concerned about my body?" Well, He's concerned enough that He mentions the word *body* 179 times in the Bible. When He deals with something that many times, it's important! The good news is that because our bodies are so important, God gives us instructions regarding how to take care of them. He tells us how we can honor Him with our bodies. Since God considers our bodies important, we should too.

God made us in His image. Wow! Think of it. It is truly awesome to have the image of the living God within us. God gave us everything we would ever need to live on this earth. Man is His crowning achievement. When man sinned and fell from grace, God gave us the best that heaven had to offer so that we could be redeemed. He gave us His only Son, Jesus. He also sent His Holy Spirit, not only to comfort us but also to indwell us. God has a huge vested interest in us, His creation. Doesn't it follow, then, that we need to take care of the bodies He has given us? Doesn't it make sense that our bodies should be finely tuned instruments fit for His use? We will honor Him by having a Bod4God lifestyle.

More Than a Weight-Loss Plan

In this book, I'm telling you how I lost more than 100 pounds. However, the book isn't just about losing weight. It's about taking small steps to change your lifestyle and put you on a path to health for the rest of your life. I call these "small steps to life." You'll move from eating food that is killing you to eating food that will build your body's strength. You'll move from being a couch potato to being physically active. You'll move from being unhealthy to being physically fit.

A very important question to ask yourself is this: "Is the way I'm living and feeling now the way I want to live and feel five years from now? Ten years from now? Twenty years from now? Is this the way I want to spend the rest of my life?" Think about how you might look and feel in a few years if you don't make changes now. Is that what you really want for your life? Do you honestly think that without making changes you will suddenly become healthy, be able to play with your kids and grandkids, put in a full day of physical activity, and be alert and engaged with others? Or do you see yourself plopped down more or less permanently in that La-Z-Boy recliner? Maybe without making changes you won't have the health issues that I had, but there are many other illnesses that are the direct result of obesity (more about that in week 9).

God says that as our days are, so shall our strength be (see Deuteronomy 33:25). As long as we are on this planet, God has work for us to do. He has much that needs to be done for His kingdom, and He is looking for those who are willing and equipped to do that work. "Equipped" means having a body that can do what He needs it to do. Moses is a great example of living a long and productive life. Deuteronomy 34:7 says, "Moses was one hundred and twenty years old when he died. His eyes were not dim nor his natural vigor diminished." There doesn't seem to be any expiration date on doing the work of God.

This book is about more than losing weight. In fact, you may not need to lose weight. If so, you are what I call a "skinny fat" person. You look like a skinny person, but your habits are those of a fat person. You were born with a high metabolism and probably couldn't gain weight if you tried. But even though you are skinny, it doesn't necessarily follow that you are healthy. This book is about how all of us can have the keys to lasting weight loss. It's about knowing what the Bible says about honoring God with our bodies. It's about how we can dedicate our bodies to God's service.

You probably have never seen me except in the beginning of this book. Even there you can see that I'm not a skinny guy, but I've come a long way toward having a fit body. I'm going to share with you my quest for lasting weight loss—a body that I can use to do God's will and live out His full plan for my life. I'm going to tell you the steps I took in acquiring lasting weight loss. I hope this book helps you do the same.

The Non-D.I.E.T. Plan

In searching for an easy way to remember the four keys that make up the Bod4God plan, I began thinking of what I had discovered as a creative way to develop a body for God. I thought about the acrostic D.I.E.T. as an effective way to remember the four keys. Those four keys, found in His Word (you will read the Scripture passages throughout this book), have helped me get to where I am now—more than 100 pounds lighter.

In the following chapters, I'm going to show you what each key is and how it can work for you. This plan is not about recording every morsel of food you put in your mouth, as many diet plans insist you do; instead, it is about making better choices about what you eat. A lot of times when we think about the word *diet*, we think about some crash plan or weight-loss program we've learned about and that other people say has been successful for them. You won't see me, or any of the others on this plan, measuring food. You also won't see us eating a lot of carbs or eating no carbs or eating only protein or eating no protein or living on grapefruit or bananas. The Bod4God Losing To Live Plan is not a "diet" plan. It is a "live it" plan!

I'm not following a short-term weight-loss program; I'm following a lifestyle program. I realize that only a small percentage of people who lose weight manage to keep it off. While it is wonderful to lose weight, it is more wonderful to keep it off. That's why the D.I.E.T. acrostic works so well. Because it is so easy to remember, what it represents encourages you to stay on the new course you have set for your life. The chart below highlights the differences between a lifestyle plan for weight loss and a short-term quick fix approach.

Lifestyle vs. Quick Fix

Long Term	Short Term
Custom Made for You	One Size Fits All
Living Food	Pills, Powders, and Potions
Ongoing Exercise Routine	Short-Term Extreme Workouts
You Enjoy It	You Endure it

In the next few chapters, I'll go into each one of these areas in depth. You will learn how to apply each key area of D.I.E.T. to your life and make it work for you for the long term. Bod4God is not about a quick fix but rather a healthy lifestyle that you enjoy living.

Self-Denial

Anorexia has never been a problem for me. Instead, as I've struggled, I've carried around more weight than God ever intended. As God began to stir in me a desire to change, I realized He needed to lead me. I asked Him to show me in His Word something that would help me build a Bod4God. I prayed, "God, give me truth from Your Word that can help me overcome this weight challenge in my life."

The passage God gave me was Matthew 16:24–25: "Then Jesus said to His disciples, 'If anyone desires to come after Me, let him deny himself, and take up his cross, and follow Me. For whoever desires to save his life will lose it, but whoever loses his life for My sake will find it.'" My weight-loss program, Losing To Live, comes from this passage of Scripture. Jesus was talking to His disciples—His followers. As believers—as followers of Jesus—this passage of Scripture is addressed to me and to you. We are the "anyone" who desires to come after Him. There's more. "Let him deny himself." You see, there is no way around it. We have to deal with self. We have to learn to deny ourselves. It requires total dedication.

Dedication by Example

When Jesus was in the Garden of Gethsemane, He prayed before going to the cross. He prayed and asked the Father, "O My Father, if it is possible, let this cup pass from Me; nevertheless, not as I will, but as You will" (Matthew 26:39). The answer to the question Jesus asked the Father was that there was no other way for salvation to be achieved. There was no plan B. It is only through His death on the cross that mankind is saved.

Jesus didn't want to die on the cross in that He didn't want to suffer the agony of crucifixion. Before He could face the crucifixion, He first had to die to self. He had to become willing to give up His life for you and me. He prayed to the Father, "Your will be done, not Mine." It took dedication for Him to die on that cross for your sin and mine. He had to deny Himself to achieve God's plan. He did it because there was no other way.

We, too, have to deny ourselves. We have to take up our cross. What is the cross in your life? For me, part of that cross was to give up bad eating habits and begin to exercise. If I wanted to follow Him, I had to deny myself in an area that was extremely difficult for me. So then, as much as we need to be willing to deny ourselves, even that much more do we need to be willing to follow Jesus's example by taking up our cross on a daily basis.

Live for Christ

Jesus instructed His disciples to deny themselves, take up their cross, and follow Him. It is in following Him that we gain true life. When we live life for self in an attempt to "save" our lives, we are sure to lose them,. Trying to save our lives has the attitude, "I'm going to live for myself. I'm going to do what I want to do." I had to stop doing that. I had to stop trying to save my life. I had to take up the cross of eating correctly and exercising. Losing my life was the only way I could ever hope to truly find it. And so I said, "Lord, I'm going to deny myself; I'm going to take up my eating and exercise cross and follow You. I'm going to *live* for You."

When you make the dedication—the commitment—to take up your cross, deny yourself, and follow Christ, life becomes exciting. Now you can begin to discover *true* life. Jesus called it "abundant life." "The thief does not come except to steal, and to kill, and to destroy. I have come that they may have life, and that they may have it more abundantly" (John 10:10). Sound good? Then quit trying to live for self. Begin living for Him and see what He can do in and through you as you begin this journey toward lasting weight loss.

My Current Lifestyle Plan

You are now on your way to developing a Bod4God lifestyle, so take a few minutes to evaluate your daily eating and exercise habits. This assessment will help you identify what "losing to live" really means for you.

My Current Nutritional Plan

How much water are you currently drinking each day?

....

....

....

....

....

Do you eat breakfast? If so, what do you eat?

....

....

....

....

What do you eat for lunch?

....

....

....

....

What do you eat for dinner?

....
....
....
....
....

What do you eat for snacks?

....
....
....
....
....

My Current Exercise Plan

Do you exercise at least three times a week? If so, what kind of exercise do you do? Fill in your exercise routine in the following chart.

Sun.	
Mon.	
Tues.	

Wed.

Thurs.

Fri.

Sat.

A Bod4God Close-Up

Small Changes Produce Big Results

Rich Kay
Lost 100 pounds

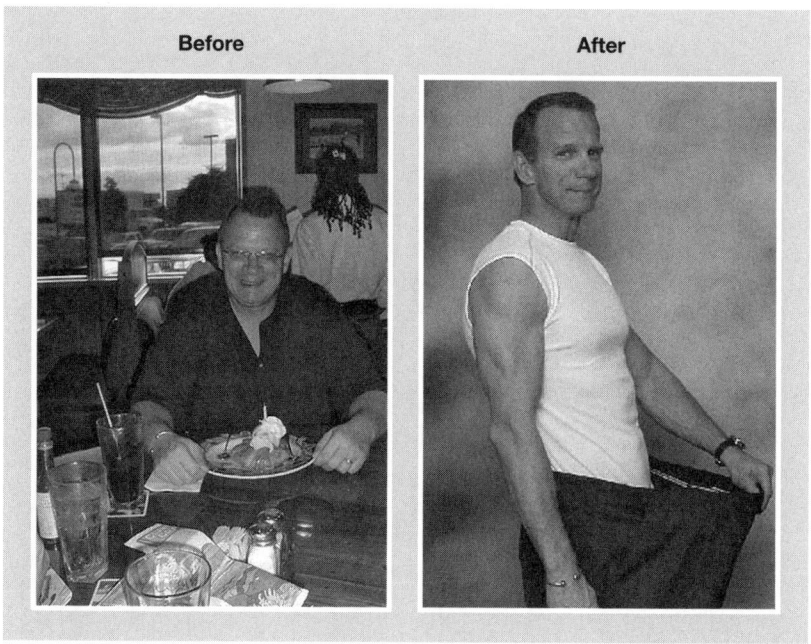

On the day I tried to roll out of bed and felt the pain and extreme effort it took to do this simple thing, I got mad, and I mean *really* mad. I looked at my body and had the following self-talk:

> What did you do to yourself, Rich? This is not you. Look at your old pictures. Just ten years ago you weighed less than 200 pounds, wore 34-inch-waist jeans, and felt okay to take your shirt off at the beach. Now you weigh 277 pounds and buy dark clothes to hide your fat rolls. Your waist size now

exceeds your age, and you are ashamed of even thinking about going to the beach without a shirt on! It's time to change. You did not gain this weight overnight, and it will take time to lose it.

That's how I began the journey. I started to take small steps to change my lifestyle, and that eventually led me to lose an average of 2 to 4 pounds a week. Some weeks I lost up to 5 pounds; other weeks I would plateau and not lose any weight, but I had faith and kept going.

I don't think I could have lost weight if I had not become angry. The battle of weight loss and weight maintenance is won or lost in your head. You, too, will probably have to get mad to make the changes necessary to lose weight. Once you reach your goal, your anger will be replaced with great confidence and self-respect, and that will keep you on track to continue the journey indefinitely. Get angry as Jesus did when the money changers were defiling His Father's house in Matthew 21:12. Jesus entered the temple courts and drove out all who were buying and selling there. He overturned the tables of the money changers and the benches of those selling doves. That's what we need to do as well.

I lost weight by doing what Pastor Steve is encouraging you to do in this book. Make small, simple changes in the way you live and see the rewards in weight loss and better health. Here's how I started:

- I got mad.
- I made one small, simple change to get to my goal: for example, I parked my car farther from my destination.
- I recorded my beginning weight: 277 pounds.

Each week I continued my small, simple changes and added some more along the journey. I started to lose weight. I continued losing weight over the next six months until I reached my six-month goal of weighing less than 200 pounds. The exciting part is I've lost more weight since then. These small, simple changes are now part of me. They are now a lifestyle. They're not a fad that I will get bored with. It is part of me. I believe that if I could do it, you can too.

I keep the weight off by continuing with a team. That has been the biggest factor in maintaining my weight loss. I have to have team support, whether it's in print, in person, or by email. I also have to keep exercising. If I go two days without physical exercise, I feel it. I call physical exercise "my little vacation." It puts me in a much better mood. We were meant to move. Even moving for a few minutes daily and building on it over time goes a long way. I didn't even go to the gym until I had lost 60 pounds. Now it is a habit. I bring my grandson with me as well. I like pumping iron, but each person has to find their own thing for exercise to keep going. Have fun with it. The key is being consistent.

Now my eating habits have changed so much that when I see a chocolate chip cookie, it looks like cardboard to me. Five years ago, if you had put a candy bar and an apple on the table, I would have eaten the candy bar. Now I want the apple.

Yo-yo dieting (gaining and losing and gaining and losing weight) is not good for a body. Focus on adding good things to your diet until they crowd out the bad foods. Instead of pursuing one diet after another, I began to replace bad foods with good ones. I've done it to the point that now I've crowded out the bad foods. My kryptonite back then was Krispy Kreme donuts. I could polish off a couple of them without thinking. Now I crave the good stuff—apples, bananas, and so on.

Food is necessary. We need it to live, but we can also easily abuse it. Our bodies are basically juice extractors. We put food in, and then our bodies extract the vitamins and minerals and dump the rest. Let's put in the most nutrient dense whole foods we can instead of the highly refined, sugar-laden, processed "Franken-foods."

Stay away from processed foods. The closer a food is to its source, the better it is for you. The more processed the foods you eat, the more possibilities there are for additives and calories you do not need. Think apple instead of an apple fritter or apple juice. If you focus on making a small, simple change a week in either eating or activity, you'll be able to maintain it. Then something magnificent happens—a snowball effect sets in. As you add more small, simple changes, the ones you are maintaining will become a regular part of your life. Once your small, simple changes are locked in, bad foods will lose their appeal.

Don't beat yourself up for not losing more weight or for falling off the wagon. Failure is not final; it's feedback. Celebrate your successes. Focus on daily achievements of moving a little more or making a healthy food choice. Take captive those negative thoughts and wrestle them to the ground. As 2 Corinthians 10:5 says, "We demolish arguments and every pretension that sets itself up against the knowledge of God, and we take captive every thought to make it obedient to Christ" (NIV).

We have to change how we think about food. We may think we deserve a reward of some kind, but it doesn't have to be food. I choose physical exercise now as a reward. Reward yourself with a smile, knowing you did well by choosing steamed veggies as a side inside of fries. Praise God for the ability to choose.

For me, temptation is not about sweets but about volume—the amount of food I eat. If I can s-l-o-w down consumption of what I'm eating, I won't eat as much. For example, at parties, food might be pushed on you. Rather than gobbling it down and soon having more food pushed on you, place some food on a small salad plate, carry it around with you all evening, and nurse it throughout the event.

The *T* for Team is essential to your weight-loss and weight-management journey. This is a team sport. In the Losing To Live groups, I focus on accountability and communication. Get folks to talk about what's going on with them. "Where are you at now?" "It's okay. You're here. You've made a decision to change. You'll get there. Remember, 90 percent of life is showing up." Did you know that those who show up more often have a higher percentage of weight-loss success? When in doubt, show up! Show up for class, exercise, the right meal choice. But show up. The team is where we can find not only accountability to keep us on track but also encouragement from one another.

Remember, when you have a bad day, start again. Never quit. What do you do when you get a flat tire? You get out and fix it. You don't get out and slash the other three tires! This too shall pass. Start again fresh the next meal or day.

During your journey to lose excess weight and improve your health, focus on making small, simple changes. Celebrate small successes. Surround yourself with a positive team. I did it, and you can do it too. *Keep moving and keep smiling.*

Note: Rich Kay's book, *Small, Simple Changes to Weight Loss and Weight Management*, is available at www.amazon.com or www.SmallSimpleChanges.com.

Small Steps to Life Ideas

What Do You Need to Know about H$_2$O?

How did you do with drinking an adequate amount of water each day? Did you follow through with it? If yes, hooray for you! If not, try again this week. It's very important to drink water. The body is 61.8 percent water. The brain is 70 percent water. We have to have water not only to survive but also to be healthy. So drink for your health!

Small Food Step

If you eat more slowly, you will consume fewer calories per meal. It takes 20 minutes for the stomach to tell the brain it's full. Train yourself to frequently put your fork down while you are eating. This gives your body an opportunity to feel satisfied before you overeat. Most of us eat so fast that we don't really taste the food. Slow down and savor each flavor. Enjoy your food, and stop eating when you're satisfied.

Small Exercise Step

Keep it simple. Just walk up the stairs rather than take the elevator. It seems like a small thing, but if a 150-pound person spends two minutes climbing the stairs, he will burn 18 calories. Want to know more? There are a number of websites where you can calculate the calories burned by the physical activities you do (a good one is http://www.healthstatus.com /calculate/cbc).

Bod4God Victory Guide

Remember that *the victory is in the Victory Guide*. Record your progress on My Progress Report located on page 22.

Week 2: Losing To Live

Bod4God Thought

Eat less and exercise more.

Bod4God Memory Verse

Then Jesus said to His disciples, "If anyone desires to come after Me, let him deny himself, and take up his cross, and follow Me. For whoever desires to save his life will lose it, but whoever loses his life for My sake will find it." (Matthew 16:24–25)

Bod4God Reflection/Application Questions

1. In Matthew 16:24–25, Jesus stated that you must lose your life in order to live. If you want to live, you've got to deny yourself. To deny yourself means total, unconditional surrender to your Savior, Jesus Christ. In what specific ways would you need to deny yourself (surrender to Christ) to improve your health?

   ....

   ....

   ....

   ....

   ....

2. How have you denied yourself and allowed Jesus to be first in your life?

   ....

   ....

....

....

....

3. If Christ is not first place in your life, what or who is?

....

....

....

....

....

4. Is your weight loss a cross in your life that you believe Jesus wants you to take up? Why do you believe it is necessary for you to do this?

....

....

....

....

....

5. What are some specific things in your life that you believe God would want you to get rid of or deny in order to improve your health and lose weight?

....

....

....

....

....

6. What are the major principles that thread through these verses? Write the principles below each verse.

Matthew 10:39

....

....

....

....

Matthew 16:25

....

....

....

....

Mark 8:35

....

....

....

....

Luke 9:24

....

....

....

....

Luke 17:33

....

....

....

....

John 12:25

....

....

....

....

7. The Bible uses the word *body* 179 times. Why do you think the Bible says so much on this subject?

....

....

....

....

....

8. What is the difference between a weight-loss plan and a lifestyle plan?

....

....

....

....

....

9. It will be important to have a support group to help you lose weight. Who are the people who will be part of your support team? Why did you choose each person?

....

....

....

....

....

10. After reading this chapter's Bod4God Close-Up, what can you relate to and what can you take from this person's story to apply to your own life and lifestyle plan?

....

....

....

....

....

Bod4God Small Steps
to Life Record

What "Skinny Things" Will You Do This Week?

Fill out this chart by indicating: (1) what you will do to eat less to live; (2) what you will do to exercise more to live; and (3) how many average daily ounces of water you will drink. Pick only a few things, and stick with them. Remember that weight loss and maintenance require you to *eat less* and *exercise more*.

Sun.	
Mon.	
Tues.	
Wed.	
Thurs.	
Fri.	
Sat.	

My Bod4God Journal

Teach me, O LORD, the way of Your statutes, and I shall keep it to the end.

Psalm 119:33

Record what God is telling you to do this week to apply the four keys to lasting weight loss.

Dedication: Honoring God with My Body

....

....

....

....

Inspiration: Motivating Myself for Change

....

....

....

....

....

Eat and Exercise: Managing My Habits

....

....

....

....

....

Team: Building My Circle of Support

....

....

....

....

D Is for Dedication

If Food Gets Near You, It Will Get in You

Walk in the Spirit, and you shall not fulfill the lust of the flesh.

Galatians 5:16

D is for dedication. Dedication is important in the challenge of losing weight. We must dedicate our bodies to God if we are ever going to have a Bod4God.

I talk to many people each week about Losing To Live. I also do many interviews on local, national, and even international radio and TV. One day a man who was at least an agnostic, and perhaps even an atheist, asked me, "Don't you think it's possible to lose weight without God?" Theoretically, I would have to admit a person can lose weight without God. People do it all the time with secular programs. However, I knew I wasn't one of them. I couldn't lose weight without God's help. I *really* needed God to guide me in this new lifestyle.

My journey began when I dedicated myself to God. In Galatians 5:16—the Scripture at the beginning of this chapter—Paul called this concept "walking in the Spirit." As the Scripture above says, when we walk in the Spirit, we will not fulfill the "lust of the flesh." What else could we call overeating and eating bowl after bowl of ice cream other than "fulfilling the lust of the flesh"? We have to call overeating and eating junk food what it is.

We have to acknowledge what we are doing before we can begin to change. I had to bring God's Holy Spirit into my life when it came to eating and exercise. I had to depend on the Holy Spirit to guide me in my choices of food. I had to ask Him to strengthen me when it came to exercise.

The Bible says that the "flesh is weak" (Matthew 26:41). That's probably an understatement. My flesh is particularly weak when it comes to eating and exercising. The Bible also says that if you walk in the Spirit, you won't fulfill the lust of your flesh. That simply means that you will allow God's Holy Spirit to control you and your intense desires for something.

In all practicality, how does this work? I was used to letting the Holy Spirit guide me when I preached, but not when I sat down to eat. I had to learn to listen for His voice prompting me to make good choices for my body—what I ate and the amount I ate. If I truly wanted a Bod4God, I could no longer stuff whatever I craved into my mouth with wild abandon. I had to stop and think about what I was about to eat.

Many of us have a gap between our beliefs and our behavior. We know what is right, but we don't do it. James said, "Therefore, to him who knows to do good and does not do it, to him it is sin" (James 4:17). I had to recognize my abusive eating for what it was—sin. I had to bring my beliefs and behavior together. For me, the first step was to dedicate my eating to God. No more playing the games of, "Well, this one bite won't hurt" or "I'll buy this treat for the kids, but I won't touch it." I had to finish with all of that. Here is the way I approached learning to honor God with my body.

Dedicate Your Body

In Romans 12:1–2, Paul wrote, "I beseech you therefore, brethren, by the mercies of God, that you present your bodies a living sacrifice, holy, acceptable to God, which is your reasonable service. And do not be conformed to this world, but be transformed by the renewing of your mind, that you may prove what is that good and acceptable and perfect will of God." In the modern Bible paraphrase *The Message*, the concept of dedication is explained a little more clearly:

> So here's what I want you to do, God helping you: Take your everyday, ordinary life—your sleeping, eating, going-to-work, and walking-around life—and

place it before God as an offering. Embracing what God does for you is the best thing you can do for him. Don't become so well-adjusted to your culture that you fit into it without even thinking. Instead, fix your attention on God. You'll be changed from the inside out. Readily recognize what he wants from you, and quickly respond to it. Unlike the culture around you, always dragging you down to its level of immaturity, God brings the best out of you, develops well-formed maturity in you.

Paul is saying, "I am begging you earnestly, dedicate your body to God!" We are to present our bodies as "living sacrifices."

Someone once quipped that the problem with a living sacrifice is that it keeps crawling off the altar. It feels that way sometimes. We can "sacrifice" for a time, but after a while we slip up, and then we either give up or have to go back to the beginning and start again.

Sometimes, dedicating ourselves to God is as simple as just saying it. "God, I give myself to You. I give my body to You for Your purposes. I can't do this on my own. I need the help of Your Holy Spirit to remind me of my calling, to encourage me when I think I can't go on and when I think things will never change." After you pray this prayer, God will help you. He can do for you what you cannot do for yourself. He can and must empower you. He can change you from the inside out. He can renew your mind. The change He can bring is not magic, but it is miraculous.

If we are not to be conformed to the world, we have to recognize the world's view of food and eating. Eating whatever you wish seems to be considered an entitlement for the majority of the American population. You work hard, and when you come home you should be able to eat whatever you wish. You've earned it. Right?

In the United States, a large percentage of people are unhealthy because they are overweight. But no wonder. Just go to a grocery store and see how much of our food didn't exist in its present form twenty or even ten years ago. There are salty chips in every conceivable shape and flavor and dozens of flavors of dips to accompany them. There are thirty-one (and many more) flavors of ice cream. There are sugared cereals by the trainload. There are sweetened soft drinks stacked to the ceiling. There are prime cuts of red meat laden with high-cholesterol fat. When you look at it that way, it's not a grocery store where you are shopping; it's a death trap—unless you learn to shop in a healthy way by shopping on the outside aisles of the store. That's where the living food is—the fruits, vegetables, dairy products, and the like. Food on the inside aisles may have been there for months.

There is a positive side to grocery shopping as well. Once upon a time, people could only eat what was in season. Now we can get fresh fruits and vegetables all year long. We have pasteurized and fortified milk and dairy products. We can buy fresh fish and chicken all year round. We are a blessed people when it comes to grocery shopping.

If we are going to dedicate our bodies to God, we are going to have to listen to the Holy Spirit's prompting every time we approach food—and that includes when we are shopping. We cannot say, "It's my body, I can do what I want with it." If you have dedicated your body to God, then it is no longer yours. So, no, you can't do what you want with it. Philippians 3:19 talks about people "whose god is their belly." Ouch! That's harsh.

Truthfully, our bellies are often all about self and doing what self wants to do. If your belly is in control of your eating and your life, you are engaging in a form of idolatry. Those of us who would never consider bowing down to a statue to worship, bow down to our appetites and make them gods. This is why the first thing I had to do to lose weight was to stop letting my belly be my god. I had to stop being an idolater. I had to admit that I had made my belly my god and then deny myself. I'm not going to pretend. It was an awful struggle; I mean really difficult.

Christians: The Most Overweight People Group in America

I said earlier that it has been determined that Christians are the most overweight people group on earth. Why is this true?

A survey by ChristiaNet reported that "out of 4,000 Christians surveyed, 39 percent did not feel that being overweight was sin. They believed that people were made in God's image, no matter their size: 'We are made after God's image, it doesn't matter how fat we are, He still loves us.' Some commented about the fact that God made each person unique and different: 'God didn't make everyone thin, and some people are just bigger than others.' Many in this category cited medical reasons or genetics for being overweight and that these reasons did not hold an individual responsible: 'Some people just can't help it, so you can't blame them.'"[1]

Such thinking may be one reason why being overweight is such a problem in our society, and particularly in the Christian community. You can shift the blame about being overweight to God by saying, "That's just the way He made me," but shifting the blame doesn't help you lose weight or improve your health.

Another possible reason is the lack of emphasis on health in most churches. I read about a study conducted by Ken Ferraro, professor of sociology at Purdue University and the director of Purdue's Center on Aging and the Life Course, titled, "Does Religion Increase the Prevalence and Incidence of Obesity in Adulthood?"[2] In an article about the study, Ferraro states that "religious shepherds need to keep better watch over their flocks and add activities to keep them from fattening up." He adds:

> America is becoming known as a nation of gluttony and obesity, and churches are a breeding ground for this problem. . . . If religious leaders and organizations neglect this issue, they will contribute to an epidemic that will cost the health care system millions of dollars, and reduce the quality of life for many parishioners.[3]

The reason I like this article so much is that right from the beginning Ferraro puts the blame squarely where it needs to go: on the pastor. I believe everything rises and falls on leadership, and I believe the main reason people are overweight in the pews is because their pastors are overweight behind the pulpit.

Ferraro also concludes that Christians accept the sin of overeating. We might preach against other things, but overeating is something we don't talk about much. "Most religions also encourage restraint from participating in injurious behaviors, such as heavy drinking and smoking," Ferraro says. "However, overeating is not considered a great sin—it has become the accepted vice." Many religious activities are rooted in food, and these foods tend to be high in fat. "These high-fat meals are saying implicitly, 'This is how we celebrate,'" says Ferraro. "Instead, religious leaders need to model and encourage physical health as an important part of a person's spiritual wellbeing."

To counter these effects, Ferraro believes that churches should encourage their members to eat healthier and engage in physical activity. He suggests organized walks with the pastor after services, serving fruit and vegetables instead of heavy casseroles at church functions, and using churches' large rooms or halls for fitness classes. "With more awareness and education," Ferraro concludes, "churches can be a positive force in fighting obesity."[4]

Like many pastors, for years I chose to ignore the problem, shift blame elsewhere, and not make my congregation aware of the importance of getting healthy. But not anymore. Now that I'm doing something about my weight and my lifestyle, I no longer have a difficult time speaking to my congregation about this problem, and no one can shift the blame to me for not addressing the issue. Paul said, "Therefore I testify to you this day that I am innocent of the blood of all men. For I have not shunned to declare to you the whole counsel of God" (Acts 20:26–27). Paul is saying, "Listen, my hands are clean. Your blood is not on my hands. I'm not responsible for your bad behavior. You can't blame me, because I preached to you all the counsel of God."

God tells us in His Word how to manage our bodies. That's part of the counsel of God. We've neglected this area in the Word of God. Do you know what God says to the pastors? "Take heed therefore unto yourselves, and to all the flock, over which the Holy Ghost hath made you overseers, to feed the church of God, which he hath purchased with his own blood" (Acts 20:28 KJV). We are to feed the flock, but that doesn't mean to feed the church of God potluck dinners. We've done a good job of feeding the stomachs of the people in our congregations. This verse, however, is talking about feeding their souls with the Word of God.

Once again, my answer as to why so many Christians are overweight is because so many pastors are overweight, and those overweight pastors have neglected this portion of the Word of God. The good news is that if the problem stands in the pulpit, perhaps the answer stands in the pulpit as well. If God will allow me, and I'm praying He will, I'm going to create a movement throughout this country and throughout the world that will get pastors and spiritual leaders on board with having a Bod4God and with preaching and teaching this truth to their congregations.

A Doctor Speaks

Dr. Liz Berbano is excited about the strides Capital Baptist Church is making toward physical and spiritual health. It matters to her, especially because she and her husband, Darren, are medical doctors.

Liz, a former lieutenant colonel in the US Army and now a staff internal medicine physician at an academic medical center in Washington, DC, has done her homework on diets and weight loss. In the health literature, the focus previously was on what diet is better and where all diets showed a benefit.[5] The question has changed from "What diet is best?" to "What motivates people to change and stick with a change?"[6] Further, research is ongoing as to which behavioral intervention can motivate someone to lose weight. Various coaching strategies have shown some benefit, but intuitively, what motivates us is highly individualized.[7]

Quoting a study in the *Journal of the American Medical Association*, Liz adds, "One way to improve dietary adherence rates . . . may be to use a broad spectrum of diet options, to better match individual patient food preferences, lifestyles, and cardiovascular risk profiles."[8] Liz believes that Bod4God is seeing success because it promotes healthy eating and exercise options and gives a spiritual reason for adherence that motivates spiritually-minded people.

Liz is also the aerobics trainer for the church's Body & Soul fitness program (more about this program in week 8). The program helps participants to become physically and spiritually fit, encouraging each other to stay with their healthy lifestyle changes as they bring God into this area of their lives. Students in the class exercise at various levels of intensity. Liz believes that because the program features music rich in biblical content, "it's nourishing for the mind and heart, as well as for the body."

Once again, remember—weight loss begins in your head and heart. I had to realize that my body was not for the gratification of self but for the glorification of God. God wants to be magnified in us. Paul said, "According to my earnest expectation and my hope that in nothing I shall be ashamed, but with all boldness, as always, so now also *Christ will be magnified in my body*, whether by life or by death" (Philippians 1:20, emphasis added).

To bring belief and behavior together, you need to apply dedication.

A Bod4God Close-Up

No Longer a Temple Trasher

Kim Wilburn-Dando
Lost 113 pounds

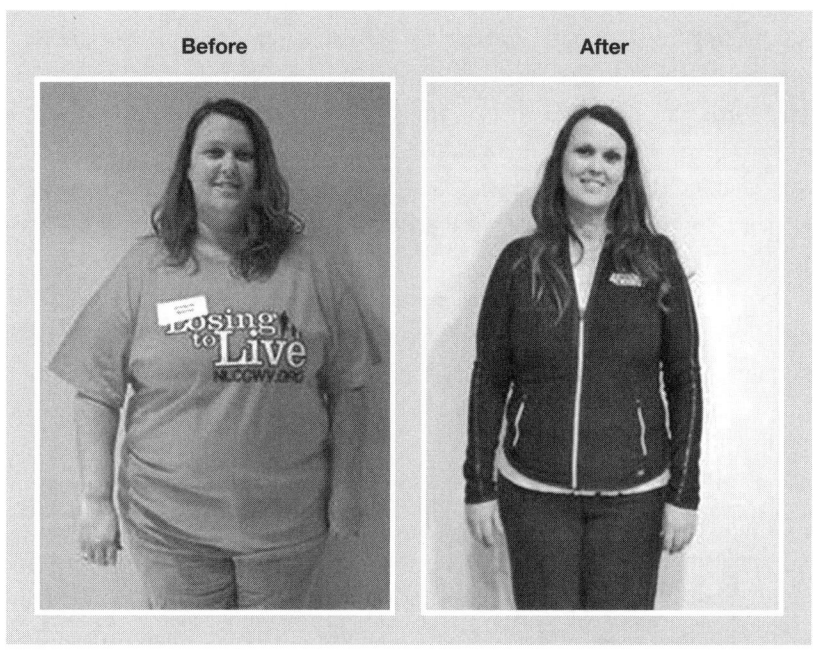

Before

After

I was very healthy growing up. I ran track and played basketball in high school, college, and in the army. Although I did not eat the healthiest diet, I remained very physically fit, ironically, until I quit smoking in my thirties. At that time, instead of turning to cigarettes to reduce stress as I had been doing, I started turning to food. I gained a significant amount of weight in a very short period of time. I also became much busier at work and made less time for physical exercise. The combination was horrific. I went from a size 5 to a size 28 over a twelve-year period of time.

Although I was ashamed of my weight gain and felt awful, I did nothing to change it.

Over those twelve years, I went from avoiding medication, even an occasional aspirin, to being on over a dozen medications around the clock for a variety of weight-related health issues. I struggled with high blood pressure, tachycardia, and had to sleep with a CPAP machine on my face because of sleep apnea. I developed COPD from many years of smoking, which was exacerbated due to my obesity. Some of the medications I was prescribed caused an increase in appetite, which resulted in weight gain. It was a vicious cycle, and I was hospitalized a couple of times for heart-related issues. Aside from the medical conditions mentioned, I was incredibly limited physically. I became unable to walk for more than 10 minutes without needing rest. My muscles would spasm, and I had difficulty breathing.

At one point, my cardiologist told me to quit investing in my 401(k), as I would not live long enough to enjoy it if I continued down the path I was on. I was upset with his statement and switched doctors, but that comment stayed with me. My pastor, Jim Goforth of New Life Community Church in Inwood, West Virginia, met Steve Reynolds at a pastors' conference in Florida. At that time, Pastor Reynolds challenged my pastor to start a Losing To Live Competition at our church. He came back excited about the *Bod4God* book, and as he spoke about it to me and others in a discipleship class and preached on it for six weeks, I was motivated to give it a try. I downloaded the book onto my Kindle and started reading it. It literally changed my life.

God gave us marvelous bodies, and we have a duty to care for them. You would not throw garbage around your church, and you should not do it to God's temple, your body. I was trashing the temple of God! I started honoring God with my body by simply adding the small steps Pastor Steve talks about. The group accountability (team) was very important. I lost 113 pounds, and my health radically improved—no more high blood pressure or sleep apnea!

My pastor's messages about honoring God with my body and being obedient to Him were my initial inspiration. Then my goal became being able to play with my grandchildren. I want to take an active role in the lives of my grandchildren for many years. Today, I also want to be as healthy as

I can so that I can take these old bones throughout the Andean mountains of Bolivia making disciples.

Initially, I focused on avoiding white flour, sugar, and soda (including diet). I also drank at least 100 ounces of water each day. Eventually, I built upon those and started including foods that provided better nourishment (grown on a plant, not made in a plant). I learned to replace things such as candy with fruit. For exercise, I literally took small steps at first. I was horribly out of shape and unable to walk for more than 5–10 minutes without having severe muscle spasms and becoming winded. So, I walked for 5–10 minutes, rested, and repeated it at least three times a day. It was discouraging at first, but once I got others to meet with me for those walks, it became easier. Teamwork was critical for me! My team was great for sharing tips, ideas, and healthy recipes, exercising together, and praying for and encouraging one another.

Bod4God: Twelve Weeks to Lasting Weight Loss and the Losing To Live Weight Loss Competition may have literally saved and probably extended my life. I was incredibly obese with multiple co-morbidities. It radically changed my life physically, medically, relationally with my family, and spiritually. A couple of months before I started the Bod4God journey, I was at Disney World with my daughter. A low point for me was when she wanted to go on a ride, and I literally could not walk up the stairs to get on the ride. She insisted and pushed me in a wheelchair up a ramp in front of a lot of people in line. I was mortified. Today, at the age of forty-seven, I am very active and pray for others I see in the condition I was in before Bod4God. I feel better, and I enjoy my life much more now that I can breathe and move more easily. I believe God can better use me for His work, which can be physically taxing.

If you are struggling with your weight like I was, I encourage you to get in a group with like-minded people and literally take the small steps suggested in this book. Once you get the hang of a few small steps, build upon them. This book teaches the importance of setting smart goals, reading labels, and reading other health and fitness materials. Most of all, pray. Pray for God to give you the desire to live healthy and to do all that is required. Don't be discouraged when you have a bad day. Just get back on track, focus on your inspiration and motivation, and surround yourself with a team that will help you in the journey. God desires for you to be healthy, and He will give you the strength to overcome the struggle if you depend upon Him to do it.

Small Steps to Life Ideas

What Do You Need to Know about H_2O?

Let's talk about water again because it is so vital to your weight loss. A good estimate of how much water to drink is to take your body weight in pounds and divide that number in half. That gives you the number of ounces of water per day that you need to drink. For example, if you weigh 160 pounds, you should drink at least 80 ounces of water per day. If you exercise, you should drink another 8-ounce glass of water for every 20 minutes you are active. When you are traveling on an airplane, because the pressurized air is so dry, it is good to drink 8 ounces of water for every hour you are on board the plane. If you live in an arid climate, you should add another two glasses per day. As you can see, your daily need for water can add up to quite a lot.

Small Food Step

By now you have probably seen a change in your weight. If so, good for you! If you have not seen a change and have been faithful in keeping the small steps, be patient; it will work in time. Let's add another small step to help you see the numbers on the scale move downward.

The only way you can lose weight is to burn up more calories than you take in. We talked about eating at a slower pace as a means of feeling full more quickly so that you can stop eating before you have eaten more than you need.

The name of the game is "portion distortion" control. A new study shows that cutting down portion size may be the single most effective thing you can do to promote lasting weight loss. Researchers found that overweight people who spent the bulk of their efforts in controlling the portion size of what they ate were more likely to lose weight and keep it off. If you are going to eat a little more of anything, make it fruits and vegetables.

Make a fist. That's about the size of your stomach. Now, be honest, if you are having weight problems, you are probably eating three or four times that much. America has become the nation of super-sized portions, and it shows in our super-sized shapes. Here are some portion sizes you need to stick to in order to lose weight:

- Meat—the size of a deck of cards
- Fish—the size of a checkbook
- Peanut butter—the size of a whole walnut
- Salad dressing—2 tablespoons
- Butter—the size of a postage stamp
- Cereal—the size of a baseball
- Rice or pasta—the size of half a baseball
- Bread—the size of one CD
- Hard cheese—the size of four dice
- Mixed nuts—the size of a golf ball

Small Exercise Step

Do two or three minutes of simple exercises when you first get up in the morning or go for a short walk outside. It will get your metabolism revved up, and that will help you burn calories all day. Continue to park your car a good distance from your office and take the stairs rather than the elevator.

Bod4God Victory Guide

Remember that *the victory is in the Victory Guide*. Record your progress on My Progress Report located on page 22.

Week Three: *D* Is for Dedication

Bod4God Thought

If food gets near you, it will get in you.

Bod4God Memory Verse

Walk in the Spirit, and you shall not fulfill the lust of the flesh. (Galatians 5:16)

Bod4God Reflection/Application Questions

1. Galatians 5:16 encourages you to "walk in the Spirit," which means to allow the Holy Spirit to control you. What does God promise to you in this verse if you will walk in the Spirit?

....

....

....

....

....

2. Is there a connection between the "lust of the flesh" and your struggle with weight? Explain.

....

....

....

....

....

3. Jesus said in Matthew 26:41, "The spirit indeed is willing, but the flesh is weak." How does Christ's statement represent your own Bod4God experience?

....

....

....

....

....

4. In what specific ways do you need to incorporate walking in the Spirit into your eating and exercise habits?

....

....

....

....

....

5. In Romans 12:1, Paul uses the word *sacrifice* when describing the dedication of our bodies to the Lord. What do you think you will have to sacrifice, or give up, in order to dedicate your body to God?

....

....

....

....

....

6. Philippians 3:19 talks about people "whose god is their belly." This verse teaches you that overeating can be a form of idolatry. What struggles have you had in this area? Explain.

....

....

....

....

....

7. As I mentioned in this chapter, I had to realize my body was not for the gratification of self but for the glorification of God. What does this mean to you?

....

....

....

....

....

8. After reading this chapter's Bod4God Close-Up, what can you relate to and what can you take from this person's story to apply to your own life and lifestyle plan?

....

....

....

....

....

Bod4God Small Steps
to Life Record

What "Skinny Things" Will You Do This Week?

Fill out this chart by indicating: (1) what you will do to eat less to live; (2) what you will do to exercise more to live; and (3) how many average daily ounces of water you will drink. Pick only a few things, and stick with them. Remember that weight loss and maintenance require you to *eat less* and *exercise more*.

Sun.	
Mon.	
Tues.	
Wed.	
Thurs.	
Fri.	
Sat.	

My Bod4God Journal

Teach me, O LORD, the way of Your statutes, and I shall keep it to the end.

Psalm 119:33

Record what God is telling you to do this week to apply the four keys to lasting weight loss.

Dedication: Honoring God with My Body

....

....

....

....

Inspiration: Motivating Myself for Change

....

....

....

....

....

Eat and Exercise: Managing My Habits

....

....

....

....

Team: Building My Circle of Support

....

....

....

....

....

D Is for More Dedication

The More You Move, the More You Lose

If you confess with your mouth the Lord Jesus and believe in your heart that God has raised Him from the dead, you will be saved.

Romans 10:9

Dedication requires discipline. From the time we are young, we hear the word *discipline* directed toward us. When we were children, most of us didn't like the word because we thought it meant punishment—time-outs, restrictions, grounding, and sometimes much more. However, discipline carries a strong positive association rather than just the negative idea we've brought from childhood. There are eleven definitions given for the word *discipline* in an online dictionary. Many of the definitions describe discipline as being the application of oneself to learning something. In fact, the most positive action definitions are "to train by instruction and exercise; drill," and "to bring to a state of order and obedience by training and control."[1]

In 1 Corinthians 9:27, Paul says, "But I discipline my body and bring it into subjection, lest, when I have preached to others, I myself should become disqualified." No matter what we are doing or learning to do, we must discipline our bodies.

Figure skaters learn the precise discipline of the required figures and spins along with complicated choreography. Competitive swimmers spend hours each day swimming back and forth in a pool, practicing the discipline of the strokes and turns while building body strength. Every sport has its disciplines. My sport was football, and I could never have played the game if I had not disciplined my body. I was on a football scholarship, and the school depended on my performance. So discipline is a good thing and something that everyone needs to practice to accomplish anything worthwhile in life.

When we talk about discipline, we are talking about something that will enhance our lives and take us to a new lifestyle. In Romans 6:11–13, Paul says:

> Likewise you also, reckon yourselves to be dead indeed to sin, but alive to God in Christ Jesus our Lord. Therefore do not let sin reign in your mortal body, that you should obey it in its lusts. And do not present your members as instruments of unrighteousness to sin, but present yourselves to God as being alive from the dead, and your members as instruments of righteousness to God.

There's that concept again—the one about losing yourself, dying to self, being dead to sin but alive to God. The "members" referred to in this Scripture passage are our body parts. The words tell us not to yield our body parts to sin. We are rather to give those body parts (all of them) to God. I finally came to the point where I disciplined all of my body parts. It has worked for me, and now I want to invite you to join me in dedicating your body parts to God. Let's make that a little more specific by starting with your feet and working upward.

Your Feet

The Bible says that feet that are dedicated to God are beautiful: "How beautiful are the feet of those who preach the gospel of peace, who bring glad tidings of good things!" (Romans 10:15). You need to dedicate your feet to God and say, "God, I want to be a witness for You, wherever my feet take me. Whether I go to church, to my job, to the grocery store or anywhere else, I want to be a witness for You. I'm not going to allow these feet to take me places that would displease You. I dedicate my feet to You for Your use and for Your glory."

So how about it, friend? Will you present your feet to God right now? If so, say, "Here are my feet, God. I give them to You for Your use."

Your Feet and Weight Loss

- Use them to exercise.
- Don't use them to walk into areas of temptation. Stay out of fast-food restaurants and any place where you are tempted to purchase or eat unhealthy food.

Your Emotions

The US Surgeon General recommends stress management as a part of the vision for the overall improved health of Americans. But even more than that, God wants us to cast our cares on Him. Therefore, we must bring our emotions under discipline. If you've ever tried a diet program before, you know that one of the first things discussed is emotional eating. Do you eat when you're stressed? When you're angry? When you're excited? One of the most detrimental emotions with regard to weight loss is bitterness. I call bitterness "frozen rage." Bitterness is a poison that can destroy your body. It is a contributing factor to many diseases. It results in depression and a feeling that life is not worth living. Your body was not designed to house bitterness. Hebrews 12:14–15 says, "Pursue peace with all people, and holiness . . . looking carefully lest anyone fall short of the grace of God; lest any root of bitterness springing up cause trouble, and by this many become defiled."

At the heart of bitterness is a lack of forgiveness. Not forgiving someone drives the issue underground where it festers and grows into a "root of bitterness." Forgiveness is not an option. It is a command: "Be kind to one another, tenderhearted, forgiving one another, even as God in Christ forgave you" (Ephesians 4:32). Choose to get better and not bitter.

Perhaps even more to the point is this Scripture passage from Matthew 6:12–15: "Forgive us our debts, as we forgive our debtors. And do not lead us into temptation, but deliver us from the evil one. . . . For if you forgive men their trespasses, your heavenly Father will also forgive you. But if you do not forgive men their trespasses, neither will your Father forgive your trespasses." The cost of not forgiving others, and allowing a root of bitterness to grow inside you, is too costly to you and to your body. You must forgive and forgive early when you have taken offense.

While reading this section of the book, you've had time to think about your own life and evaluate if an unforgiving attitude and a root of bitterness are affecting your ability to change your lifestyle so that you can lose weight. Are you ready to change? Are you ready to make a commitment to forgive and pull out your root of bitterness? If so, say, "God, I want to present all my emotions to You, especially my bitter attitude."

Your Emotions and Weight Loss

- Keep your stress level low through prayer, exercise, and reading God's Word.
- Remember that resentment only punishes you.
- Don't use food as a medication—as emotional eating.
- Remember that the Bible says, "Be anxious for nothing" (Philippians 4:6).

Your Hands

You might ask, "What do my hands have to do with losing weight?" The Bible says, "Cleanse your hands, you sinners" (James 4:8). Think about what you do with your hands. I used my hands to pick up the wrong kind of food and put it in my mouth. Perhaps for you, it's not just food but cigarettes or marijuana or many other things that are detrimental to your health and well-being. Perhaps it's using your hands to touch someone who is not your spouse. "Cleanse your hands, you sinners."

Let's dedicate our hands to God to do His work. Hands are an active part of our Bod4God. "God, I'm going to honor You with my hands. I'm going to please You with my hands."

Your Hands and Weight Loss

- Use them to grab a bottle of water.
- Use them to detox your kitchen.
- Move them to select healthy foods and prepare healthy meals.

- Don't use them to pick up chocolate.
- Don't use them to pick up unhealthy food.

Your Mouth

The mouth (which includes the tongue) may be the most difficult body part of all to bring under discipline. I'm not talking here about what goes into your mouth as much as what comes out of it. Learning to discipline the tongue and what you say will take you a long way toward a lifestyle change. James warned us:

> Even so the tongue is a little member and boasts great things. See how great a forest a little fire kindles! . . . But no man can tame the tongue. It is an unruly evil, full of deadly poison. With it we bless our God and Father, and with it we curse men, who have been made in the similitude of God. Out of the same mouth proceed blessing and cursing. My brethren, these things ought not to be so. (James 3:5, 8–10)

Of course, in a book about weight loss, we have to talk about disciplining ourselves concerning what we put into our mouths as well as what comes out. Proverbs 23:1–2 says, "When you sit down to eat . . . put a knife to your throat if you are a man given to appetite." That's pretty severe! God doesn't actually want us to cut our throats to prevent us from overeating, but He's trying to tell us, "Hey, overeating is serious because it destroys your health." This Scripture passage is telling us to take drastic action to control overeating.

I always say, "When you love potlucks more than you love God, you have a serious problem." When "all you can eat" is the way you live, you need discipline. If you are prone to gluttony, you need to take drastic measures to bring your appetite under control. I'm a man given to appetite. Therefore, I have to take drastic measures to control what goes into my mouth.

Will you give your mouth and what comes out of it as well as what goes into it to God for His use? "God, here's my mouth. I'm giving it to You."

Your Mouth and Weight Loss

- Use it to pray and ask for God's help.
- Use it to eat healthy food.

- Use it to encourage others to eat in a healthy way.
- Don't use it to speak negatively to yourself or others.

Your Eyes

King David said, "I will set nothing wicked before my eyes" (Psalm 101:3). There is a lot we could say about movies, TV shows, and internet pornography and near-pornography that come into our minds through our eyes. More than ever, and because of such easy access to these kinds of visual stimulation, we have to discipline our eyes. Turn off the TV. Don't go to websites that exist only to pollute your mind. Choose media and entertainment wisely. Set no wicked thing before your eyes.

When we're talking television and weight loss, what about all the television advertisements for food products that do not enhance good health? There are thousands of products advertised on TV that are not healthy. Then there's the Food Channel, where someone is cooking delicious-looking meals nonstop, 24/7. Yes, a few of them are promoting healthy eating, but not enough to warrant keeping the channel on all day long. We have to discipline our TV viewing.

Let's all make this commitment: "God, help me keep my eyes pure, and show me if I'm causing others to stumble in this area."

Your Eyes and Weight Loss

- Use your eyes to read God's Word and encourage yourself.
- Use them to read helpful information about good health.
- Use them to look in the mirror and think positive things about yourself.
- Use them to enjoy the beauty of the healthy foods God has created.
- Don't use them to watch the Food Channel or too much TV—get moving instead.
- Avoid the lust of the eyes, which includes focusing on unhealthy foods.

Your Ears

With the advent of smartphones and many other ways to access audio information and music, we need a rededication of our ears to God. Keep them pure and listen to what will help you grow as a believer. James 1:19 says, "Be swift to hear, slow to speak." Above all, learn to listen with your inner ear to the voice of the Holy Spirit as He tries to guide you toward great choices that will make you a healthy person with a Bod4God.

From a weight perspective, just think about all the information about food that comes to us through our ears. We are bombarded with talk about food, not only from the media but also from any small group of people standing around chatting. Much of the time, their conversation is dominated by talking about food. We have to resist the temptation about food that comes to us through our ears.

Think about this: Eve fell into sin when she heard what the serpent said about the forbidden fruit and was encouraged to eat it. He challenged her with, "Has God indeed said, 'You shall not eat of every tree of the garden'?" (Genesis 3:1). Eve listened. She listened, she heard, she disobeyed, and she ate the fruit. Let us not listen to the temptation that comes through our ears.

Let's dedicate our ears. "God, help me to be a listener to good things."

Your Ears and Weight Loss

- Use them to listen to praise music—while you exercise.
- Use them to listen to good advice from others.
- Use them to listen to God's voice.
- Use them to listen to information that will bring better health.
- Don't listen to words like "Just a little won't hurt you."

Your Mind

The Bible says, "Let this mind be in you which was also in Christ Jesus" (Philippians 2:5). That's a huge goal, and we will spend the rest of our lives striving to have the mind of Christ by surrendering our thoughts to Him in all things.

We protect our minds from evil when we discipline the rest of our body parts. If we don't allow evil to come into our minds through our eyes, ears, mouths, and hands, we are protecting our minds. That's half the equation. The other half is learning how to access the mind of Christ. How would He think about certain things?

Several years ago, there was a popular campaign in the Christian community asking, "What would Jesus do?" It's still a valid question. One way to know how Jesus would think and act is to stop before acting and ask that question: "What *would* He do?" Of course, in order to know the answer to the question, we need to be reading the Word of God. It has all the answers for life, and it will tell us what Jesus would do in any given situation.

The standard for our thought lives is Philippians 4:8:

> Whatever things are true, whatever things are noble, whatever things are just, whatever things are pure, whatever things are lovely, whatever things are of good report, if there is any virtue and if there is anything praiseworthy—meditate on these things.

Make a new commitment to discipline your mind. Say, "God, take my mind and set it on things that bring You glory."

Your Mind and Weight Loss

- Think about God.
- Allow Christ to renew your mind on a daily basis.
- Use your mind to research and gather new information on health.
- Think about what you are eating.

Your Heart

Last of all, discipline your heart. Just how do you do that? Romans 10:9 says, "If you confess with your mouth the Lord Jesus and believe in your heart that God has raised Him from the dead, you will be saved." First, you have to dedicate your heart to God through forming a relationship with Him. You have to become a follower of Jesus Christ. The way to do this is to realize you are a sinner and have broken God's laws. The Bible says that because we have broken His laws, we deserve eternal death and hell. But Jesus, the sinless Son of God, came to earth, died on the cross for our sins, was buried, and rose from the grave to give us eternal life through Him. To be forgiven and have eternal life, we must follow Romans 10:9 above. Confess and believe, and you will be saved. It's so simple that many people miss it.

Discipline comes when we make sure that what our lips say and our hearts believe are the same. Jesus talked about people who honor Him with their lips, but their hearts are far from Him. If you have never confessed Jesus Christ as your Lord and Savior and come to believe in Him as the only one who can save you from both the penalty and the power of sin, then your lips and your heart are in two different places. Here's the way to make the commitment to bring them together:

> *Dear God, I'm a sinner. Because of my sin, I deserve to spend eternity in hell. I believe Jesus died on the cross, was buried, and rose from the grave for my sins. I turn from my sins and put my faith in Jesus Christ to get me to heaven. Thank You for saving me today, and help me to serve You the rest of my life. In Jesus's name I pray. Amen.*

Your Heart and Weight Loss:

- Accept Jesus Christ as your Savior and Lord.
- Don't let a root of bitterness grow in you; cultivate a heart of forgiveness toward others.
- Love God with all your heart.

This is the end of week 4 on your journey to better health. I hope that you have dedicated yourself, your life, and your body to God and are ready for the next step in the process. In order to achieve lasting weight loss, you must continue on and find the inspiration you will need to sustain you and keep you focused on your goal.

A Bod4God Close-Up

Spiritual Healing That Led to Physical Healing

Ana Sufitchi
Lost 80 pounds

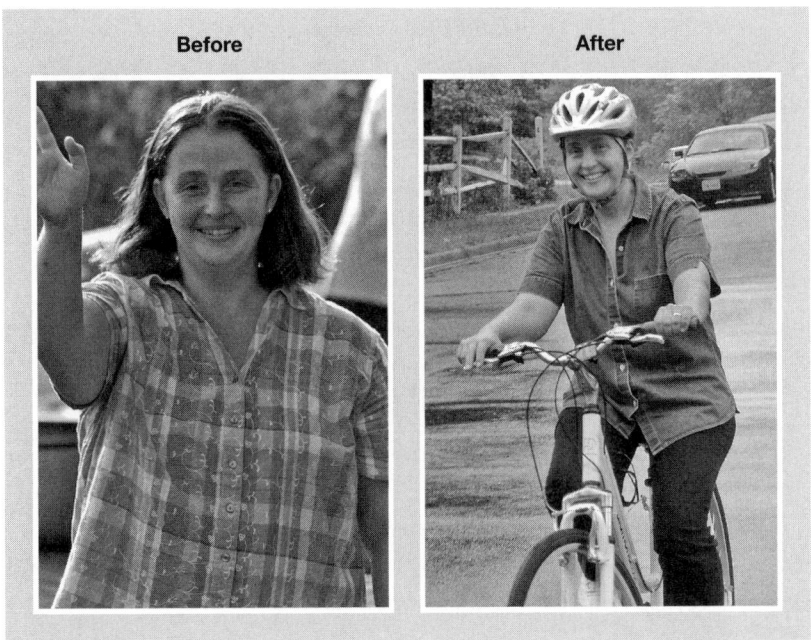

Before **After**

I was born in Romania, and my family moved to the United States in 2002. I was active and enjoyed hiking in the mountains of Romania during any type of weather, and I loved to play in the waves of the Black Sea regardless of the size or the strength of them. I had many wonderful experiences; however, some decisions that I made brought me more stress than I could handle. This stress took its toll on my health and sent me to the operating room five times in five years. It also caused problems with some of my relationships.

I needed something in my life, and that something was Jesus. I respected God, but I did not have a personal relationship with Him through Jesus Christ. But He wanted me, so He brought me to my knees and broke my will in many ways. Out of this brokenness I asked Jesus Christ to be my Savior and Lord. At this time, I was taking my body down a dangerous path that included a series of different illnesses, and I was carrying an unhealthy amount of weight. In His mighty mercy, God began my restoration process. In the same way that a wonderful stained glass window is built out of thousands of broken pieces, my inside and outside started to change and rebuild. I am not a finished work, and God is still molding me every day. However, giving God my complete trust and having faith in Him to lead my life from all points of view allows me the freedom to be courageous and dream with boldness.

After my salvation and after I offered myself completely to God, little by little, my healing started, a process that amazed my doctors. I have been able to lose 80 pounds. My love for my husband, kids, and parents has been my inspiration. I realized that if I didn't change my lifestyle and model it after God's Word, my life would be headed in a dangerous direction, negatively impacting all of my loved ones.

Our bodies are the temple of the Holy Spirit. *Temple* is a word that we don't use very often in our daily language. We attend worship services in a building that we call a church. How would you feel if you saw somebody behaving without care on your church property or, even worse, inside the sanctuary? Aren't our bodies more important to God than a building? Our bodies are wonderfully made, crafted with care for each of us. God sent the Holy Spirit to live in us, and our earthly bodies are His home. Ask yourself, am I taking care of God's home, my body, in a way that makes Him happy? Am I using my body as a real witness for Christ? These are questions that helped me get closer to the root of the Bod4God lifestyle.

So what helped me lose the weight? The answer is the Losing To Live Weight Loss Competition at Capital Baptist Church in Annandale, Virginia. Here I learned to take small steps to life. I started drinking water and eating a healthy breakfast, and I incorporated green vegetables into my meals at least once per day. I also started participating in exercises that I loved, like swimming, fast walking, biking, and gardening. I try to exercise at least twice per week. To maintain my motivation and to challenge myself,

I register for competitions like 5K and 10K walking races. This forces me to prepare for a challenge that will occur relatively soon in my life, which helps keep me in shape. I still struggle with stress management; however, eating right and exercising help with this.

I have read *Bod4God: Twelve Weeks to Lasting Weight Loss* with passion a few times. I even translated it with help from my father into my native language, Romanian, because I needed to plant deep in my heart the seed of my new Bod4God lifestyle. The Losing To Live Weight Loss Competition is part of my lifestyle, helping me to stay strong even in my weaknesses related to eating and weight management. It helps me with accountability and encouragement, provides friendship and comradery, provides prayer support, and offers valuable information and advice. It also deepens my relationship with God through the Bible study that we do and helps me control my emotional eating. Emotional eating is a problem for many. I have had to learn to make peace with myself and with others, to ask others for forgiveness and to forgive as the Lord forgave me. There is peace for a troubled heart, and once you have peace, mindful and responsible eating is much easier to achieve.

As Christians, our mission is to serve the good of others and to be a witness of our wonderful faith in Jesus Christ to the world. This mission is almost impossible to accomplish in poor health. That is why it is so important for us as Christians to maintain our health to the best of our ability. I urge you to schedule some quiet time with God and in a very honest way ask Him if your lifestyle, your attitude toward your health, and your body make Him happy. If they don't, ask Him to help you change. In a humble way, ask God to help you take care of yourself according to His Word.

This is the story of my Bod4God lifestyle, how I adopted it, and how I am determined to continue it for the rest of my life. I have experienced many ups and downs. I learned how to keep close to God and Losing To Live, especially during the hard times, like weight-loss plateaus, temptations, or even peer pressure. Bod4God is a lifestyle that you need to adopt for the rest of your life.

Small Steps to Life Ideas

What Do You Need to Know about H$_2$O?

In addition to making healthy nutritional choices and exercising daily, drinking adequate amounts of water is extremely beneficial for weight loss. Avoiding dehydration is crucial if you are trying to lose weight. This is true for several reasons, but one of the most pertinent factors has to do with water's effect on the body's vital organs. Studies have shown that a low consumption of water allows more fat to be deposited instead of being metabolized into energy. Water helps our kidneys flush out toxins. The kidneys cannot perform their function properly without water, and this forces the liver to assist with water filtration. The result is interference in the liver's primary function, which is to burn fat. So drink a sufficient amount of water!

Small Food Step

Nobody can keep to a totally restrictive diet that never allows for a treat. Just make sure that your "treats" are healthy, such as fat-free yogurt sprinkled with a few nuts, strawberries dipped in a tiny bit of melted dark chocolate, a cup of melon pieces, or a few pretzels—not the whole bag.

Small Exercise Step

Anyone can find thirty minutes a day for exercise. Here are some ways:

- Give up one TV sitcom rerun and exercise instead. Or get a treadmill and walk on it while you watch TV.
- Walk while listening to podcasts or audio books on your smartphone. It will make your walk time seem shorter.
- Walk to errands or appointments rather than take the car.
- Work around your house—indoors or out. Housework and gardening can burn quite a number of calories.

- Chase a kid. Babysit for a young mother or a single parent who needs a break. It helps you and it helps them. Toddlers never sit still, so you'll have to chase them around to keep them out of trouble.
- Get a dog and walk it.

Bod4God Victory Guide

Remember that *the victory is in the Victory Guide*. Record your progress on My Progress Report located on page 22.

Week Four: *D* Is for More Dedication

Bod4God Thought

The more you move, the more you lose.

Bod4God Memory Verse

If you confess with your mouth the Lord Jesus and believe in your heart that God has raised Him from the dead, you will be saved. (Romans 10:9)

Bod4God Reflection/Application Questions

1. How would you state this week's memory verse, Romans 10:9, in your own words?

   ....

   ....

   ....

   ....

2. Has there ever been a time when you dedicated your heart and life to Jesus Christ? Describe this event and the way it changed the way you live.

   ....

   ....

   ....

   ....

   ....

3. Take some time to think about your body and your health while the information you have just read is fresh in your mind. What steps do you plan to take to change each part of your body? List these in the chart below.

Body Area	What steps do you need to take in relationship to your health to dedicate this area to God?
Feet	
Emotions	
Hands	
Mouth	
Eyes	
Ears	
Mind	
Heart	

4. Within the context of weight loss, which of your body members are most difficult to discipline?

....

....

....

....

....

5. Why do you think this area is such a struggle for you?

....

....

....

....

....

6. The title of this book, *Bod4God,* is used throughout the text. Now that you have completed this part of the study, what does the term "Bod4God" mean to you?

....

....

....

....

....

7. After reading this chapter's Bod4God Close-Up, what can you relate to and what can you take from this person's story to apply to your own life and lifestyle plan?

....

....

....

....

....

Bod4God Small Steps to Life Record

What "Skinny Things" Will You Do This Week?

Fill out this chart by indicating: (1) what you will do to eat less to live; (2) what you will do to exercise more to live; and (3) how many average daily ounces of water you will drink. Pick only a few things, and stick with them. Remember that weight loss and maintenance require you to *eat less* and *exercise more*.

Sun.	
Mon.	
Tues.	
Wed.	
Thurs.	
Fri.	
Sat.	

My Bod4God Journal

Teach me, O LORD, the way of Your statutes, and I shall keep
it to the end.

Psalm 119:33

Record what God is telling you to do this week to apply the four keys to
lasting weight loss.

Dedication: Honoring God with My Body

....

....

....

....

Inspiration: Motivating Myself for Change

....

....

....

....

....

Eat and Exercise: Managing My Habits

....

....

....

....

....

Team: Building My Circle of Support

....

....

....

....

....

I Is for Inspiration

Short-Term Pleasure Is Not Worth Long-Term Pain

The thief does not come except to steal, and to kill, and to destroy. I have come that they may have life, and that they may have it more abundantly.

John 10:10

Most of us know that we need to get healthier. The problem is that we're not motivated to do anything about it other than talk about it; and once in a while we get started and then give up within a week or two when we are not satisfied with the results. In this chapter, we're going to talk about how to get motivated and stay that way. Weight loss is about a lifestyle change, and it won't happen unless you are inspired to take those first steps and then stay with the program.

Some of us become inspired when the doctor tells us that if we don't lose weight we're going to lose our lives. Some of us get sick of not being able to tie our shoes without huffing and puffing over a big stomach. Some of us have an event to attend for which we want to lose weight. It doesn't matter what the inspiration is, the important part is to find out what works for you and get going on a plan.

To encourage you, let me remind you that by making Small Steps to Life in your diet and exercise routine, you can begin to reduce your waistline. It isn't complicated. It isn't costly. But it does take determination and commitment, and lots of it.

Your Body Was Created for God

Let me remind you once again that your first inspiration must be that your body was created by God and for Him. God gave you life. God sustains your life. God is the one keeping your heart beating and your brain functioning.

God cares about our bodies. He cares if we are healthy or not. I believe this, and it's why my church and I are on the front lines of the fight against fat. It's also one of the reasons the media is so interested in what we are doing. It's a new concept to many people that God cares about our health. Many journalists who interview me are merely looking at the physical side of things. This fight, however, is also a spiritual battle. The enemy of our souls is as interested in us being overweight, without energy and unhealthy, as God is in us being at the right weight, having energy and becoming healthy. We are not going to be our most effective in God's kingdom if we cannot function at peak physical efficiency.

Where Can We Find Inspiration?

The first question of the Westminster Shorter Catechism confession of faith is "What is the chief end of man?" The answer is "To glorify God and enjoy Him forever." If we are to glorify God, can we do it with a body given over to gluttony? Can we glorify Him with a body that we've failed to consider is His abode on earth? So how do we come to the place where we are inspired to face this giant of a challenge in our lives and begin to take steps to slay it so that we can glorify God and enjoy Him forever?

In a joyous burst of enthusiasm, the apostle Paul writes, "Now may the God of hope fill you with all joy and peace in believing, that you may abound in hope by the power of the Holy Spirit" (Romans 15:13). And the writer of Hebrews declares with great joy, "Look unto Jesus, the author and finisher of our faith, who for the joy that was set before Him endured the cross, despising the shame, and has sat down at the right hand of the throne of God" (Hebrews 12:2).

The Bible contains the inspiration we need for all the challenges of life, including the challenge of losing weight. For me, Matthew 16:24–25, with regard to denying myself, taking up my cross, and following Jesus, was a huge inspiration for change. I had to realize that life wasn't going to be easy as I began to deny myself. I was going to have to lose a favorite part of my life—eating lots of food. Then I began to realize that giving up the overindulgence of food was the only way for me to find my life. That was very exciting!

God gave me Matthew 16:24–25 to encourage me. I knew I wanted to experience the fullness of life in Christ. I wanted to be a fit tool for His use. I wanted to be well and happy and live to see my grandchildren and maybe even my great-grandchildren. I wanted to find my life, and here in this verse, I found out how to do it—deny myself, take up my cross, and follow Him.

Simple . . . and very difficult to do. But there's good news on that front. The Bible says, "I can do all things through Christ who strengthens me" (Philippians 4:13). Christ is so pro-life that when you set out to do something difficult like getting a Bod4God, He's right there to help you live.

There's a war going on between the Lord Jesus and Satan over you and your body. Satan doesn't want you to succeed in weight loss or anything else that will make you more effective for God. Satan is a thief who will rob you of good health. He'll do everything he can to discourage you. In John 10:10, Jesus says, "The thief does not come except to steal, and to kill, and to destroy." But there's good news in the rest of the verse. Jesus says, "I have come that they may have life, and that they may have it more abundantly."

Abundant isn't a word we use too often these days, but we should use it when we are talking about God's goodness and grace and His ability to help us. The dictionary definitions of the word *abundant* will bless your soul. It means "present in great quantity; more than adequate; over-sufficient, well supplied, richly supplied." He's got everything you need for a new life—one that works for Him, one that is able to do His will, one that is eternal.

I realized the thief was coming into my life through too much food and too little exercise. Satan was stealing from me. I had diabetes, and diabetes can kill you. Satan was killing me with a knife, fork, and ice-cream spoon, and I wanted to live. I wanted to receive the promise Jesus gave—the promise of living life more abundantly. What I wanted was a better quality of life and a better quantity of life. I had to lose myself so that I could live. That's what inspired me—the desire to live.

Be Inspired to Live and Impact Your Family

I want to be on earth as long as I can to be with my family and impact their lives. I have an amazing wife named Debbie. I want to be around to enjoy old age with her. God has blessed us with three wonderful married adult children. I am so proud of Crystal and Bakary, Sarah and George, and Jeremiah and Carria. I am also a grandpapa! Olivia, Salima, Camden, and Kaitlyn (and hopefully more to come!) bring me indescribable joy. I want to see them grow up and make an impact for God.

I don't know what my legacy will be at the church. That's up to God. I am most concerned, however, about the legacy I am leaving my family, and I want it to be a positive one. My hope and prayer is that God will allow me, through living a healthy lifestyle, to live a very long life and be around for my family. I want to be here to love them, support them, and influence them.

When it comes to wellness, I want to be a good example for them. I want them to see me eating a healthy diet, exercising, and taking care of my body. In the past, I did not set a good example for them. I was digging my grave with a knife, fork, and ice-cream spoon. But now I've taken the steps needed to have a Bod4God.

I am truly looking forward to going to heaven, but I am not in a hurry to get there. The truth is I need my family, and they need me. Your family needs you too. I encourage you to honor God with your body and live.

Be Inspired to Give a Good Account to God

One day we are all going to stand before God and give an account of our lives. Romans 14:10–12 says, "But why do you judge your brother? Or why do you show contempt for your brother? For we shall all stand before the judgment seat of Christ. For it is written: 'As I live, says the LORD, every knee shall bow to Me, and every tongue shall confess to God.' So then each of us shall give account of himself to God."

The big things for which we'll give an account include:

- Our *time*. We all have the same amount of time (twenty-four hours in a day), and we're going to have to answer to God for how we used our time.
- Our *talents*. What did we do with the talents God gave us?
- Our *treasure*. We'll have to answer to God about our money and how we used it.
- Our *temple*, what we did with our bodies. One day you are going to deliver your body to God and say, "God, here I am, standing in judgment before You." God's going to shine His light on your time, talents, and treasure, and He will also look at your temple.

In 2 Corinthians 5:10, Paul writes, "For we must all appear before the judgment seat of Christ, that each one may receive the things done in the body, according to what he has done, whether good or bad." Will you be able to give a good account to God?

An Inspiring Story of Overcoming Addiction

If you eat more than your body needs, you are addicted to food. Several years ago, a wonderful story was told in the Condensed Book section of a *Reader's Digest* magazine about a Baptist pastor. His name was Gordon Weekley, and he was in a hurry to build his church and congregation in his church-planting endeavor. His people responded to his inspiring messages as they, along with Gordon, envisioned what their church would be like.

Soon the church needed two Sunday morning services. He became busier and busier, and his wife only saw him at bedtime, and his children even less. On a visit to his physician, he explained that while life was going well, he sometimes felt a little jittery. Weekley was having trouble falling asleep once he finally crawled into bed. The doctor prescribed something to "help him sleep."

It worked and he slept deeply and woke refreshed until a little later in the day when the anxiousness returned. He didn't worry, as he knew he would sleep that night. Then the pills didn't work so well, and he began to take one and a half and then two. He stopped eating supper, thinking that maybe the pills would work better on an empty stomach. He started losing weight.

Along the way, he started taking another drug to help him feel peppier after having taken the drug that made him able to sleep. He was glad for the extra energy as he cared so much about his church and his people. He wanted to be everywhere at once, but he didn't know if it was because he loved them or because he wanted to be loved.

Finally, his physician realized just how many prescriptions his office was writing for him and told Gordon to go get checked out at the hospital. Gordon went willingly, all the while saying, "I can stop taking the pills any time I want." But he couldn't, and his life spiraled downward rather quickly.

It was his wife who first tried to call him to accountability, but he would have none of it. His denial was so deep that he could not admit he was a drug addict, and without that admission, nothing could change. Finally, his wife had had enough. She packed her bags, took his four sons, and left. He went to his study and wrote a letter of resignation to the church he'd worked so hard to build.

Life went from bad to much worse as he wandered from family member to family member and then on to friends and finally to wandering the streets in a drug-induced stupor. At last, a friend called on the phone and confronted him. "Gordon, this thing has been going on a long time. You've tried everything, and nothing has worked. I think there is one thing you haven't tried. You haven't tried God."

Of course, Gordon denied this vehemently. He said he had prayed and asked God for help—over and over again.

"But," his friend persisted, "have you ever really, truly, given this over to Him? Recommit yourself. Pray with me now."

His friend prayed for this poor lost man and asked God to return him to the fold. Gordon hung up the phone, went to his bedroom, and went down on his knees. There, he admitted that he couldn't handle his own life anymore and that he wasn't getting better. He put himself in God's hands and then rose and went to bed. He fell asleep knowing that he had come to the end of himself and couldn't "fix" it this time. It was out of his hands.

Gordon didn't see any visions that night—he just went to sleep—and in the morning, he opened his eyes and saw only the ceiling of his bedroom.

Something had changed in him, however: he felt no anxiety. He knew that he would be facing another day without pills, but he suddenly felt no desire for them. He felt calm, refreshed, and at peace.

It's so utterly simple, Gordon thought. *I've preached it over and over, and I still didn't see it. "Put yourself in God's hands." How could I have missed it all these years?*[1]

That was the miraculous end of Gordon Weekley's terrible addiction. While we may not believe that our addiction is as serious as his, it might well be. God is available to deliver you from your food addiction in the same way he delivered Gordon. Think hard about the way in which Gordon Weekley stopped denying that he had a problem, put himself in God's hands, and then rose and went to bed. He rested in God's ability to do the work in his life that he could not do. That same power is available to deliver you.

A Bod4God Close-Up

Jesus, My Drill Sergeant

Robert Clyde Lockley
Lost 85 pounds

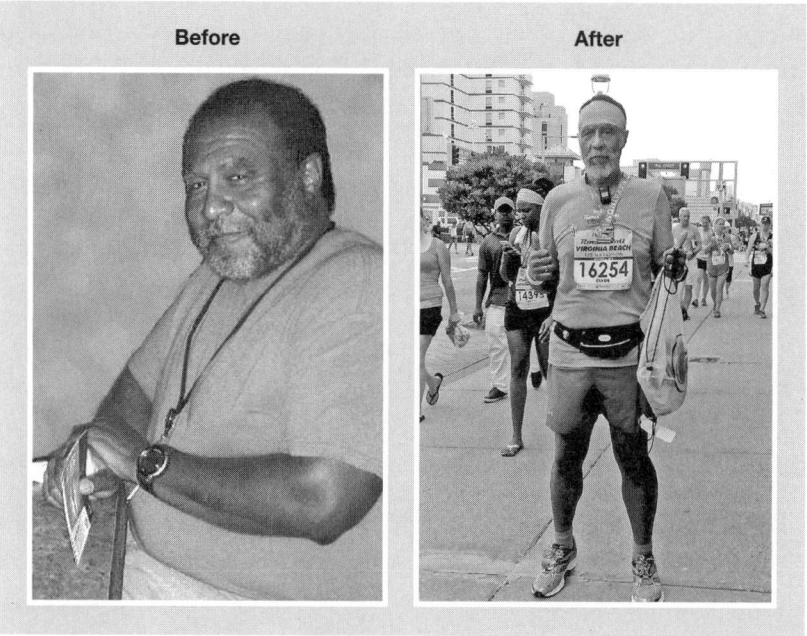

Before

After

After graduating from high school, I joined the army and loved everything about the military. I worked and exercised hard and ate very well, and the army kept me fit. When I became a drill sergeant, I knew I had hit pay dirt, and I loved keeping my soldiers fit by training with them. Calling cadences for double time or marching was my specialty. I was in the best shape of my life.

Upon completion of my military service, I kept the same eating habits, did little to no exercise, and didn't have any soldiers to train with. As you can imagine, I started to gain weight, and I got larger and larger. My doctor put me on three blood pressure medications, I had borderline high cholesterol, and my blood sugar levels were elevated. At 300 pounds, I was sick and could do very little about it. I finally realized that my health was not good and my life was in danger.

One day I heard Pastor Steve Reynolds on the radio and my life changed. It was in January of 2013 when I heard him say, "Don't lose weight alone; join a team of losers." That statement began my lifestyle change. My challenge was to overcome more than twenty-five years of struggling with being overweight and unhealthy. I was skeptical about the program, but God got a hold of me. Even though I had never heard of people getting off blood pressure medication because of weight loss, I thought, *What do I have to lose?*

Once I was introduced to Pastor Steve and the Losing To Live Weight-Loss Program, I learned to focus on the fact that I am the keeper of the temple that God has loaned to me and taking care of my body is a spiritual act of worship to God! I meditated on Romans 12:1, which says, "I beseech you therefore, brethren, by the mercies of God, to present your bodies a living sacrifice, holy, acceptable to God, which is your spiritual service." I started the process of losing weight to shed about 30 pounds, but not long into the process, it became less and less about losing weight and more about getting healthy and honoring God with my body. Through this spiritual revelation, God allowed me to see what I was doing to my body and what kind of example I had become. This was the moment that everything changed, when I was able to let go of the past and move forward in living a healthy life.

Thank God I have been able to lose 85 pounds, and I now weigh around 220 pounds, which is within 10 pounds of what I weighed at my high school graduation. I was able to achieve this goal by making small steps to life in eating and exercising, such as drinking water and green tea, incorporating more foods that grow from the ground into my diet, and making homemade smoothies from healthy foods. I discovered that a person can get filled up eating fiber and not be hungry and, therefore, not overeat. I learned that sacrificing your likes for a short period of time can help your taste buds change, and when they change, everything else will change.

When I was looking for small steps to life in exercise, I knew I had to find exercises that I enjoyed and could consistently do. So I started walking every day, bicycle riding, swimming, taking the stairs (not the elevator), walking up escalators, and doing repetitions of very light weights. I enlisted the help of a personal trainer. I realized that the more weight I lost, the easier it was for me to exercise. Since I had a lot of weight to lose, I started slowly, but as I lost weight, I was able to exercise more.

I could not have made this incredible transformation on my own. My Losing To Live team has been a great help. I received lots of encouragement from them. During times when I did not lose any weight, they helped me figure out how to get past it and move forward. I was so impressed with the results from my first Losing To Live session that I participated in the program two more times at Capital Baptist Church in Annandale, Virginia. I have taken the program back to my former church, the Upper Room Fellowship Church, and became a co-leader at my church, South Potomac Church, because I know it works. I want others to experience the same success I had.

The most important part of my team is my wife. After I had lost 30 pounds, she became interested in what I was doing. I never suggested that she should lose weight. She saw with her own eyes the healthy changes I had made and the results I had achieved, and she became interested in weight loss. It is such a blessing to me to have her by my side as we continue this journey of a healthy life.

This program is your program. Once you dedicate your body to God, incorporate healthy lifestyle changes, and start praising God, your emotions and whole outlook on life will start to change. I also want to encourage you to pray to God to help you get rid of any bitterness you might have toward others, even if it is from years ago. Holding on to bitterness is like taking cyanide and expecting some other person to die. Let go of the painful things from the past and start moving forward toward a better, healthier future.

I want to encourage you to surrender to God and join a team of losers. You must attend meetings regularly, stay connected to your team, and build your healthy lifestyle program. Pastor Steve Reynolds says we need to "become a student of fitness and nutrition," and I want to pass that advice on to you. The process of changing your health and wellness is not easy. My unhealthy eating habits and sedentary lifestyle were not easy to uproot, but the Losing To Live program helped to change my desires to what God wanted them to be. If I can do this, anyone can.

Small Steps to Life Ideas

How are you doing? Have you memorized any of the weekly Bible verses? If you have, you can meditate on them when temptation comes calling and when it just seems too hard to go on. That's important, so keep trying to memorize a verse a week. Now for some more small steps to add to those that have worked successfully for you.

What Do You Need to Know about H_2O?

We are still talking about water because it is so important. Did you know that if you have a mere 2 percent drop in your body's water supply, it can trigger fuzzy short-term memory, trouble with basic math, and difficulty focusing on smaller print such as that on a computer screen? Mild dehydration is one of the most common causes of fatigue. For the most part, the majority of the population is going around somewhat dehydrated, and this is in a country where all we have to do is turn on a tap for clean water. It doesn't make sense, does it?

Small Food Step

Detoxify your kitchen. If you haven't done so yet, go through your cupboards and refrigerator and get rid of every snack and food that is unhealthy. There are those of us who cannot have food items like ice cream, peanut butter, packages of cookies, chips, etc. You know where your weakness is. Dump it—and don't go dig it out of the garbage later when you're hungry. It's a simple fact that if you don't have junk food in your house, you are much less likely to eat it.

Small Exercise Step

If you like riding a bicycle, do it now. It's a great way to develop muscle, burn fat, work your heart, and get that metabolism up. Oh, and it can be a lot of fun too. And then, if you're out in the sunshine, you're soaking up that vitamin that suddenly everyone is talking about and recommending—vitamin D. Don't forget to wear a helmet and keep to safe bike paths. If you have a bike but aren't ready to get outside and ride in front of everyone, you can get a bike stand that turns your bike into an exercise machine.

Bod4God Victory Guide

Remember that *the victory is in the Victory Guide*. Record your progress on My Progress Report located on page 22.

Week 5: *I* Is for Inspiration

Bod4God Thought

Short-term pleasure is not worth long-term pain.

Bod4God Memory Verse

The thief does not come except to steal, and to kill, and to destroy. I have come that they may have life, and that they may have it more abundantly. (John 10:10)

Bod4God Reflection/Application Questions

1. In John 10:10, John tells us that Satan wants to destroy us. He steals from us and attacks us during our weakest moments and in our weakest areas. When you examine your own health issues regarding weight, where does Satan attack you, and what is he stealing from you?

....

....

....

....

....

2. When Jesus states that He came to give you an abundant life, this includes your health. What part of your health/weight do you think the Holy Spirit would have you change to live abundantly?

....

....

....

....

....

3. You will have to give an account to God for how you use your time, talents, treasure, and temple. What specific things do you need to do now to prepare for this final judgment?

....

....

....

....

....

4. In Matthew 21:12, Jesus got angry and drove out the greedy money changers from the temple because they were not respecting it. Similarly, 1 Corinthians 6:19 states that your body is the temple of the Holy Spirit. Are you angry at Satan's influence over your eating and exercise habits and the negative impact it is having on your health? Explain your answer.

....

....

....

....

....

5. Look up the following verses. How could each verse motivate you when the going gets rough?

Proverbs 16:3

....

....

....

....

....

Jeremiah 32:27

....

....

....

Romans 6:6–7

....

....

....

1 Corinthians 6:12

....

....

....

Ephesians 6:11

....

....

....

....

Philippians 3:13–14

....

....

....

....

....

6. There is power in God's Word. Do you have a Bible verse that you have claimed for maintaining a Bod4God lifestyle? If so, what is it? If not, find a verse that you can claim for your victories and recite when temptation surrounds you. Write the verse below.

....

....

....

....

7. What is your motivation for losing weight?

....

....

....

....

....

8. After reading this chapter's Bod4God Close-Up, what can you relate to and what can you take from this person's story to apply to your own life and lifestyle plan?

....

....

....

....

Bod4God Small Steps
to Life Record

What "Skinny Things" Will You Do This Week?

Fill out this chart by indicating: (1) what you will do to eat less to live; (2) what you will do to exercise more to live; and (3) how many average daily ounces of water you will drink. Pick only a few things, and stick with them. Remember that weight loss and maintenance require you to *eat less* and *exercise more*.

Sun.	
Mon.	
Tues.	
Wed.	
Thurs.	
Fri.	
Sat.	

My Bod4God Journal

Teach me, O LORD, the way of Your statutes, and I shall keep it to the end.

Psalm 119:33

Record what God is telling you to do this week to apply the four keys to lasting weight loss.

Dedication: Honoring God with My Body

....

....

....

....

Inspiration: Motivating Myself for Change

....

....

....

....

Eat and Exercise: Managing My Habits

....

....

....

....

Team: Building My Circle of Support

....

....

....

....

....

I Is for More Inspiration

What You Eat in Private, You Wear in Public

I can do all things through Christ who strengthens me.

Philippians 4:13

One huge reason why people fail when they set out to lose weight is because they have unrealistic goals for weight loss. Of course, magazines and television, weight-loss camps, and a host of other unrealistic information sources cause us to believe that you set out to lose weight and it just falls off. You've probably discovered that's not true. And when we don't reach the unrealistic goals we've set, we become discouraged and reach for the chips and dip to dull our discouragement.

We have to get real. Even if we lose weight, most of us are not going to look like the models in magazines or even the people in weight-loss ads. First of all, those images have probably been computer enhanced and you wouldn't recognize the models if you met them on the street. So let's set some realistic goals about how we will look when we lose weight. We have to learn to accept our bodies. When you lose weight, you won't suddenly have blue eyes and curly hair—unless you had them before you lost weight. You probably won't have fabulous six-pack abs even if you exercise a lot. But you will look better than you do in your overweight condition, and you will definitely feel better. So get real about what losing weight is going to do for you.

Here are some things to keep in mind when you are trying to reach a weight goal:

- Action drives motivation.
- If you step on the scale and see no weight loss (or perhaps only a little), remember that it took you a while to gain all this weight and it will take time to lose it. It will happen if you stick to your goal of creating a Bod4God lifestyle.
- Take a look back and see how far you've already come. And remember that even if you are not losing weight this week, if you're not gaining any, you are making progress.
- If you miss exercise one day or eat something you know will not help you reach your goal, get back on track the next day or the next time you eat.
- Spend a few minutes remembering that a worthwhile payoff lies ahead. You will be an improved you.
- Remember all the benefits of exercise over and above weight loss, such as the fact that it improves mood, combats chronic disease, helps manage weight, strengthens the heart and lungs, and promotes better sleep.

Setting Goals

Someone once said that if you don't set a goal, how will you know where you are going and how will you know when you arrive? And when you get back, how will you know where you've been? It is important to set a goal and it is important to keep that goal in front of you. Write down your weight-loss goal on a sticky note and post it on your bathroom mirror. Post it in the front of this book. Post it on your computer screen or on the dashboard of your car.

Setting a goal tends to focus you on what you want to achieve. It's like a contract with yourself. It drives your motivation. Keep the goal achievable. Set your goal realistically so that you can be successful. That will keep you motivated. Here are some tips for goal setting:

- Write down your goal. Post it where you will see it often.
- Make the goal attainable. "I will lose 1 to 2 pounds a week."
- Let everyone know about your goal and get people to encourage you. Spouses and children are notorious for trashing weight-loss plans. Explain to them what you are trying to achieve, a Bod4God, and ask them to be supportive.
- Vary your exercise and try to have fun. Take a walk one day, lift weights the next, ride a bike, swim, or play basketball or handball. Watching TV while moving your body can help take the tediousness out of exercise and give you something to look forward to during that time.
- Try new seasonings and flavors in your food but stay away from any that add calories. There are tons of recipes online for healthy, delicious dishes that will bring new flavors to your palate. Type "weight-loss recipes" into an internet search engine for more healthy food ideas than you will live long enough to eat. Go to the Mayo Clinic website and type in the search box "weight-loss recipes" and you will find an expansive list, including main dishes, appetizers, and even desserts. In addition, I highly recommend First Place 4 Health as an excellent resource for healthy recipes.
- Reward your success on reaching your goal, but don't do it with food. This is one of the toughest places to retrain yourself, because most of us have been rewarded with food from the time we were sitting in a high chair.
- Remember the Scripture, "I can do all things through Christ who strengthens me" (Philippians 4:13).

Four Spiritual Motivators for Change

1. Rely on God

The number one way for me to stay motivated is to rely on God. There is no way I could have achieved my goals without the help of the Lord. When I rely on Him, I am not alone. He is with me. As I've already said, many people contact me about my weight loss and about our Losing To Live Weight Loss Competition. I make it a priority to talk to them because I want to learn what is going on in their lives. I try to connect what is happening in their lives with the culture in which they live. I want to know others' struggles so that I can make this message practical and relevant to readers.

When Jesus's disciples fell asleep in the Garden of Gethsemane rather than staying awake with Him to pray, Jesus said to them, "Watch and pray, lest you enter into temptation. The spirit indeed is willing, but the flesh is weak" (Matthew 26:41). That admonition was not just for those sleepy disciples; it's for all of us who seek to improve our bodies for God's use by losing weight. Even though I knew for a long time that I needed to get healthy and needed to lose weight and exercise, my spirit was willing, but my body wouldn't cooperate. One of the functions of the Holy Spirit is as a helper. I had to learn to pray specifically for the power of the Holy Spirit to fill my life and help me. I had to learn to walk in the Spirit—at the dinner table, in my recliner after dinner, and at church functions where there was an overabundance of food. I made a conscious decision to walk in the Spirit on those occasions. What went for the eating part of the equation also went for the exercise part. The Holy Spirit had to help me get moving. I literally had to "move" with the Holy Spirit.

2. Refine Your Attitude

One of the first things I had to do to achieve a Bod4God was to refine my attitude. The Bible says, "As he thinks in his heart, so is he" (Proverbs 23:7). In other words, "Your attitude, not your aptitude, determines your altitude in life." I had some unhealthy attitudes to work through before I could rise above my weight, and perhaps you do too.

Do you reject your body? Some of us look at our bodies and say, "God, You messed up when You made me." Most overweight people suffer from low self-esteem. For some people, it starts in childhood when they are presented with Ken and Barbie dolls. I decided that my girls were not going to have Barbie dolls. I didn't want them to have an impossible-to-achieve shape as a model for what they should look like when grown. My son didn't have Ken or G. I. Joe dolls either. Those male counterparts to Barbie are as ridiculously unachievable as the female dolls. I certainly have never looked like either Ken or G. I. Joe. When I was growing up, I looked more like Mr. Potato Head or the Pillsbury Dough Boy.

With regard to your body, the important thing to remember is that God gave it to you. And no matter how much you try to change it through weight loss or surgery or exercise, you are still stuck with the basic framework you got when you were born. The best thing you can do is learn to love your body, treat it well, and realize that while it's not perfect, it is the temple of God.

The key here is balance. We are to love and care for our bodies, but not make them idols that consume our thinking and our time. Remember, God says that we are "fearfully and wonderfully made" (Psalm 139:14).

3. Read the Bible Every Day

I can't emphasize enough that the Bible is the recorded Word of God given to us. It is a "living word" that brings health and vitality to our inward life. It's the way we renew our minds. It's the way we get to know the Author and His Son. It provides the encouragement we need to put off our former lifestyle and take up a new one. Ephesians 4:23 says, "Be renewed in the spirit of your mind." That's it. Feed your mind with healthy thoughts just as you feed your body with healthy food.

In addition to reading the Bible, meditate on it. Think about what you are reading. When you were little, your mother told you to chew your food thoroughly. (That's still good advice for weight loss. It helps you feel satisfied with less food.) The same goes for God's Word. Chew on it. Extract the meaning. Apply what you read to your own life. Make decisions based on what you've read and learned.

Joshua gave this instruction to God's people: "This Book of the Law shall not depart from your mouth, but you shall meditate in it day and night, that you may observe to do according to all that is written in it. For then you will make your way prosperous, and then you will have good success" (Joshua 1:8).

4. Read Health-Related Books or Materials Every Day

There are thousands of books and magazines on health, diet, and exercise. I'm a busy guy and I don't have time to read lots and lots of stuff. But every day I try to read some kind of health-related material to feed my mind a little bit and get me thinking about what I need to be thinking about. We have a model in Paul. In 2 Timothy 4:13, Paul asked Timothy to "bring the cloak that I left with Carpus at Troas when you come—*and the books, especially the parchments*" (emphasis added). The parchments were the Word of God, but it appears that Paul had an interest in other kinds of good books.

Hosea 4:6 says, "My people are destroyed for lack of knowledge." Today, there is no excuse for anyone to have a lack of knowledge—about anything, much less about health issues. We are in the middle of the greatest explosion of knowledge the world has ever seen. Information can go around the world with the speed of light. Go to the internet and put in any health-related issue you can think of and up will come hundreds of sites where you can get information. Of course, you have to be careful about what kind of information you are accessing and using, because anyone can post anything he or she likes on the internet and some of what shows up there is useless and even dangerous information. Once again, rely on the Holy Spirit to guide you to the best sources of information.

Bookstores have huge sections crammed with health-related and weight-loss information, or you can go to the public library for a lot of free health information.

There are at least a dozen health-related magazines that have current and updated information with every issue. The same cautions you use to access internet sites apply to choosing books and magazines to read. Be careful what you put into your mind. Choose that which "renews" the mind.

What to Do with This Knowledge

What should you do with all the knowledge you've gained through reading this book and others? Start to put the information into practice. No more *mañana* (tomorrow) diets. No more Monday diets—you know the ones: KFC on Sunday complete with chicken skin, mashed potatoes, and gravy with the justification, "Tomorrow morning, baby, no more mashed potatoes and gravy for me. I'll kick it into high gear once I get beyond this last fling."

Once I got serious, I knew I had to start my healthy eating on Sunday or whatever day comes before *mañana*. No more excuses. No more procrastination. James 4:17 says, "To him who knows to do good and does not do it, to him it is sin." So what you do with your newly acquired knowledge is to put it to work creating a better body for God. Stop making the wrong choices. Stop making excuses. Start today to become a better you.

If You Are Still Asking Why You Need to Change

You will have to recognize that this is going to be a fight. You will get hungry. You will get lazy. You will want to give up. That's the time to remind yourself why you are doing this at all. Remember:

- You'll feel better.
- You'll have more energy.
- You'll have fewer pains.
- You'll look better.
- You'll gain strength spiritually.
- You'll live as if your body is the temple of God.

You can't give up when things get tough. You have to hold on to whatever it is that is inspiring you to change and to achieve the lasting weight loss that you desire. The results will be worth it in the end. Now that we have the dedication and inspiration down, it's time to move on and discuss eating and exercising.

A Bod4God Close-Up

Living a Happy, Heart-Healthy Life

Gail Mates
Lost 70 pounds

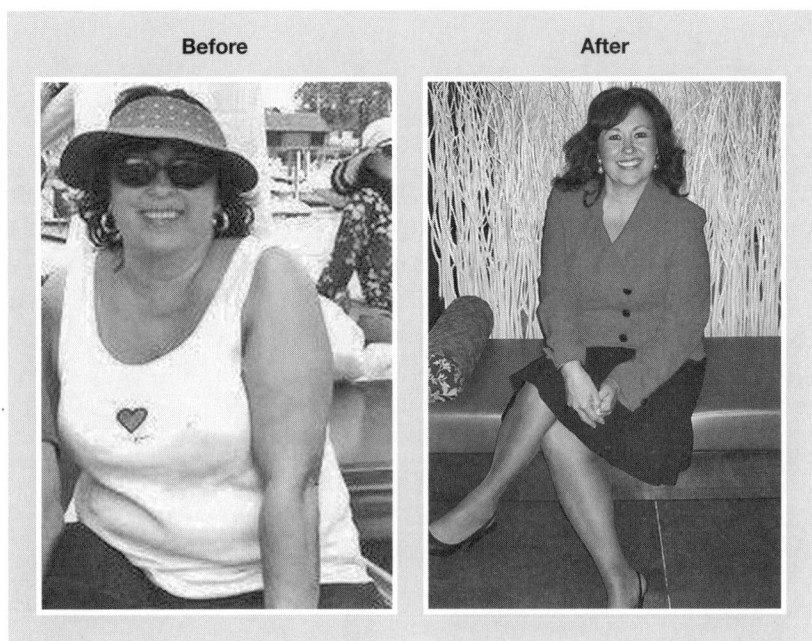

One of my biggest struggles with weight loss stems from when I was a child. I was overweight for most of my life. My mother wanted me to be slim, and in the second grade she put me on a diet. Mom's putting me on a diet only made me want to eat more. Ultimately, food became my comfort, something that I worshiped. I lived to eat, and my eating was definitely emotional. When disappointment would enter my life, I would go into my closet and not only eat but eat in despair. I learned to medicate myself with food as opposed to facing my issues and struggles.

My family also has a bad tradition of heart disease. Almost everyone in my family has died from it, and I was the next in line. When my father had two heart attacks and then a stroke from which he died, I became very depressed. I didn't care if I lived or died, and I was eating uncontrollably trying to dull the pain with food. This resulted in my developing many risk factors for heart disease. I had diabetes, high cholesterol, high blood pressure, a waist circumference much bigger than 35, metabolic syndrome, bleeding ulcers, asthma, and sleep apnea. I also needed esophagus surgery.

My physical health was so bad that my daughter would come into my room in the middle of the night to see if I was still breathing. She said to me, "With your family history of heart disease, you are killing yourself, and you will not be around for me and your future grandchildren." She was eighteen when she said this to me, and it was at that time I knew I needed to make a change. I happened to see an advertisement for the Losing To Live Weight Loss Competition at Capital Baptist Church in Annandale, Virginia. I called the church and actually spoke to Pastor Steve Reynolds, and after I shared my story with him, he said to me, "You are missing a team of people to help you lose weight." So I joined the program, and after dedicating my body to God and taking small steps to life, I started to lose weight. Pastor Steve was right. I needed the team to support and listen to me, and I needed to listen to the advice and encouragement they provided me. We reached out our hands together to embrace a Bod4God lifestyle. The most important person on my team was God, and I could pray to Him often with faith that He heard my heartfelt prayers of wanting to change my life and live.

I have learned to face my fears and disappointments by talking them over with my team instead of engaging in emotional eating. I set goals each week for small steps to life. I started with five minutes of exercise a week and slowly increased it. I felt so triumphant and empowered when I was able to do more and more. Then I was able to achieve a lifelong goal of completing a 5K race/walk. I proudly participated in the Losing To Live 5K with my family cheering me on. I also completed a 10K race with a teammate.

Through the program I have lost over 70 pounds, and all my health problems and risk factors are gone. Because my transformation was so dramatic, I was chosen out of thousands of women to be a national spokesperson for the American Heart Association. I have even been featured on an

NBC nationwide TV special on my lifestyle changes, spurred on by Steve Reynolds's *Bod4God* book. I am especially proud of the American Heart Association's Lifestyle Change Award that I received. I now represent the Centers for Disease Control's Million Hearts Campaign for the prevention of heart disease. God has taken me on an incredible journey as I share my story with others around the country.

I often think back to that little girl struggling to lose weight and be thin. It was an obsession. Today, I just want to be healthy. I don't have to hide from anyone anymore. It wasn't the big changes I made that helped me lose weight but rather the small steps. It was the power of God that changed me. I have learned that the team approach makes all the difference.

I have been given a new lease on life, and I am blessed and thankful for the *Bod4God* book. If it weren't for this program, I would not be living a happy, heart-healthy life. You have to believe in God and yourself, and you have to have a team supporting you. This program saved my life and also made my faith in God stronger. Prayer works, and having a Bod4God lifestyle will give you the dedication, inspiration, and motivation you need to lose the weight and keep it off. Live the life that God intended for you to live and bring a vitality and vigor into your life through an increased relationship with Him.

Small Steps to Life Ideas

What Do You Need to Know about H₂O?

Additional considerations for drinking an adequate amount of water include the following:

- Water assists in absorption, digestion, and metabolism of food because our bodies' proteins and enzymes work more efficiently in diluted solutions.
- Drinking lots of water results in more muscle mass because our muscles are composed primarily of water.
- Water gives us the energy and hydration needed for exercise.
- When adequate amounts of water are not consumed, our bodies hold on to excess water for survival, causing bloating.

Small Food Step

Eat with people who have small appetites and observe how they eat. They probably put their fork down between bites. They probably have only one small serving of the foods they eat. They may turn down dessert, but if they are served dessert, they will probably take only a couple of bites. After all, the first bite tastes the best. At the same time, don't eat with people who encourage you to overeat. Probably some of those people are overweight. Fat friends support each others' bad eating habits. They too are toxic to you.

Small Exercise Step

Remember that muscle burns calories even when the body is at rest. It's something like the idling engine of a car. A car doesn't burn as much fuel in neutral, sitting in the driveway, as it does running at 70 miles per hour down the highway. Your muscle won't burn as much fat when you are resting, but it burns something. That's better than nothing. Get that muscle growing.

Bod4God Victory Guide

Remember that *the victory is in the Victory Guide*. Record your progress on My Progress Report located on page 22.

Week 6: *I* Is for More Inspiration

Bod4God Thought

What you eat in private, you wear in public.

Bod4God Memory Verse

I can do all things through Christ who strengthens me. (Philippians 4:13)

Bod4God Reflection/Application Questions

1. Paul believed he could do all things through the strength of Jesus Christ. Do you really believe that Christ will give you the strength to maintain a Bod4God lifestyle? Why or why not?

....

....

....

....

....

2. How will you apply this to your life this week? Read the passages in the following table and summarize each in your own words. Then go back and put a check mark next to verses you find inspirational.

John 10:10	
Philippians 4:13	
Colossians 1:16	
Psalm 139:14	

Matthew 16:24–25	
James 4:17	
Galatians 5:16	
1 Corinthians 6:19–20	

3. Proverbs 23:7 says, "As he thinks in his heart, so is he." Are you experiencing a balance between rejecting and perfecting your body? Explain your answer.

....

....

....

....

....

4. Why do you think the motivation to live a healthy lifestyle is often so difficult?

....

....

....

....

....

5. What is your motivation for losing weight? To live longer? To look better? To feel better? Or something else? Explain your answer.

....

....

....

....

....

6. After reading this chapter's Bod4God Close-Up, what can you relate to and what can you take from this person's story to apply to your own life and lifestyle plan?

....

....

....

....

....

....

Bod4God Small Steps
to Life Record

What "Skinny Things" Will You Do This Week?

Fill out this chart by indicating: (1) what you will do to eat less to live; (2) what you will do to exercise more to live; and (3) how many average daily ounces of water you will drink. Pick only a few things, and stick with them. Remember that weight loss and maintenance require you to *eat less* and *exercise more*.

Sun.	
Mon.	
Tues.	
Wed.	
Thurs.	
Fri.	
Sat.	

My Bod4God Journal

Teach me, O LORD, the way of Your statutes, and I shall keep it to the end.

Psalm 119:33

Record what God is telling you to do this week to apply the four keys to lasting weight loss.

Dedication: Honoring God with My Body

....

....

....

....

Inspiration: Motivating Myself for Change

....

....

....

....

Eat and Exercise: Managing My Habits

....

....

....

....

Team: Building My Circle of Support

....

....

....

....

....

E Is for Eat

Eat for Your Health, Not Your Happiness

Each of you should know how to possess his own vessel in sanctification and honor.

1 Thessalonians 4:4

You've probably heard the adage that if you fail to plan, you plan to fail. You can have all the goals in the world, but if you don't have a plan to reach them, you'll never reach your goals. In this chapter, I want to help you discover and create a feasible plan to achieve whatever goal God has placed on your heart.

Maybe you don't know what your goal should be. James 1:5 says, "If any of you lacks wisdom, let him ask of God, who gives to all liberally and without reproach, and it will be given to him." Whenever we are in a quandary, we can ask God for wisdom. I challenge you to do so as you create a plan to achieve your goal. Ask God to lead you. There are many plans to weight loss, and sticking to a plan is the key to success.

Choose a Plan That Is Best for You

One of the main reasons most people fail on traditional diet plans is that they are told to eat what other people choose for them to eat. This approach simply doesn't work for most people because we don't all have the same appetites, background, or circumstances. Bod4God is about crafting your own plan that you will do gladly for the rest of your life.

Get a Multitude of Counsel

Start talking to people about all the options for weight loss so you can figure out what will work best for you. Listen to what worked for them. Read the weight-loss stories in this book. Consider how to adapt the program those successful losers used to your specific concerns and needs. Get input on your plan from lots of sources. This is a biblical concept as well. Proverbs 15:22 says, "Without counsel, plans go awry, but in the multitude of counselors they are established."

Don't Wait to Make Your Plan: Do It Now

Advance decision-making is critical to a healthy lifestyle. Yet another proverb has really helped me here. "A prudent man foresees evil and hides himself, but the simple pass on and are punished" (Proverbs 22:3). Healthy living requires foresight.

My life is busy, and I have to set a plan. If I don't plan ahead, any goal I have set for myself doesn't happen. Not too long ago, I went to a pastors' conference. I knew it would be held at a nice, fancy hotel where there would be a lot of food. I can't say I was perfect in sticking to my healthy living lifestyle, but I did pretty well. I knew I was going to be breaking my routine. I had to think, *You're going to have less control over food choices. Think about how you're going to deal with those potatoes when they're put in front of you. What are you going to do with them?* I exchanged them for salads. I usually decide what to order at a restaurant before going in. This helps me to deal with a tempting menu.

Follow a Routine

When you start making changes, your body will probably resist change at first. If you get on a routine, your body will get used to it. Make healthy eating a major part of your routine. Eat smaller portions and let your body get used to less food.

Think about the law of sowing and reaping in relationship to your health. Galatians 6:8 says, "He who sows to his flesh will of the flesh reap corruption." If you sow to your flesh by eating anything you want to eat, and if you don't exercise, you're going to corrupt your body. But if you sow to the Spirit, you will reap life. Galatians 6:9 encourages us by saying, "Let us not grow weary while doing good, for in due season we shall reap if we do not lose heart."

It is important to encourage yourself, because when you begin to make changes, it is very hard to follow through. Those first few weeks and days are difficult. Be encouraged that repetition will train your body to perform new habits and crave new things. If you hang in there, you can retrain your body for lasting weight loss.

I love what Paul said in 1 Corinthians 9:27: "I discipline my body and bring it into subjection." I have to train my body, and the good news is that when I do, a lot of the things I used to crave I no longer want. For example, when I woke up this morning, the first thing I craved was an apple and a glass of water. It hasn't always been that way. But now, around lunchtime, I crave a salad because most days I eat a grilled chicken salad for lunch. When I began my Bod4God quest, it was about meat and potatoes and, of course, ice cream. It was about as little exercise as possible. Now, I've found a plan and a path that work for me, and I'll never go back to the lifestyle I once had.

Making a lifestyle change with regard to what you eat demands some thought and study. The very foundation of building a healthy lifestyle is realizing that God gave you life and a body and that you're to take your life and body and please Him in the things you do with them. Since there are so many mentions of the body in the Bible, we can know for sure that God didn't leave us on this earth without direction as to how we should manage our bodies. Matthew 16:24–25 states it plainly: to gain your life, you have to lose it. I had to become a loser, and that's where the Losing To Live idea came from. We can't take the easy way out. We have to eat less and exercise more—it's that simple.

We know what we should do to have better health. It's self that gets in the way of doing it. Self wants to eat the foods that are not healthy. Self doesn't want to exercise. Self doesn't want to die daily. But it's the only way we can lose to live.

Obey the Bible

The secret to weight loss is that there is no secret. You simply have to eat less and exercise more. You have to face this reality and quit looking for a pill or a potion to solve your weight-loss need. So let's talk about the issue of managing your habits. Again, the Bible comes to the rescue. The main verse that has helped me here is 1 Thessalonians 4:4: "Each of you should know how to possess his own vessel in sanctification and honor." In the beginning, I didn't know how to "possess" my own body—I didn't know how to manage it. I had to learn. We can all do better about the way we eat. We can all improve. But how? How do we make choices that are healthy? How do we learn what is best for us?

Proverbs 4:20–22 is helpful: "My son, give attention to my words, incline your ear to my sayings. Do not let them depart from your eyes; keep them in the midst of your heart; for they are life to those who find them, and health to all their flesh." The place to start with lifestyle changes is the Bible—the Word of God. There are two basic things that the Word of God teaches with regard to losing weight and having a healthy lifestyle. Here they are.

1. Eat in Moderation

For me, and for many of us who are overweight, eating in moderation means eating less. For all of us it means making healthier eating choices. For someone who is anorexic, it means eating sensibly—the right things in the right portions to keep the body healthy. When I was overweight, Proverbs 23:2 always bothered me because it says, "Put a knife to your throat if you are a man given to appetite." I used to quickly skip over this verse, first because I didn't really understand it and second because I didn't like knives, particularly around my throat. But then I started to think about what it really means and realized that it is speaking about gluttony and how seriously we need to take overeating. The writer of this proverb is telling us to take action and to change our eating habits. Remember, your stomach is the size of your fist, so you do not need to eat portions the size of your head.

2. Get the Right Amount of Exercise

Overweight people don't want to hear that they need to exercise. We blame a low metabolism for an inability to lose weight, and it is probably true for many of us. But some of you are skinny and you have terrible eating habits. You are sneaking by because you have a high metabolism. While many overweight people envy you, you too may be a glutton. (Tough talk, huh?) I'm not a scientist or a nutritionist, but I know we can't use slow metabolism as an excuse to be overweight. We have to get our bodies moving. We have to exercise to get our metabolism going. If you do enough exercise and eat less, you will very likely lose weight. God always intended for us to move and be physically active. Genesis 2:15 says, "The LORD God took the man and put him in the Garden of Eden to tend and keep it." From the very beginning, God expected us to work and be physically active.

How Then Shall You Eat?

The answer to what shall we eat is simple: *better* and *less*. Eat less and eat foods that are as close to the way God made them as possible—straight from the ground, straight from the trees. Eat food for health and not because you think it will make you happy.

God is one cool God. He created food, and He wants us to enjoy our food. He put ten thousand taste buds on the tongue, in the throat, and in the esophagus that provide information about the taste of the food we eat. Taste buds detect the four elements of taste perception: salty, sour, bitter, and sweet. The food we eat hits clusters of these taste receptors, which transfer the information to the cortex of the cerebrum in our brains. It's a complicated process that was given to us for one reason. God wants us to enjoy the taste of our food.

Food is beautiful—especially food in its natural state before all identity has been processed out of it. I suppose God could have made all our food gray in color and it could have been just as nutritious as it is now, but He didn't do that. He made orange food—carrots, pumpkins, and citrus fruits. He made dark green leafy vegetables, some with red stems to appeal first to the eye and then to the palate. He made foods that are red and purple and white and yellow, and they are beautiful, and we want to eat them. Go to a store that specializes in fresh fruits and vegetables—a place like Pike Place Market in Seattle, Washington, where fruits and vegetables are stacked on farmers' tables like works of art, or a Whole Foods store found in many major cities where there are lovely piles of fresh food. Or visit a farmers' market or roadside stand in season and just enjoy the sight of the beautiful food God has given us in its natural state. God wants us to enjoy the way our food looks.

The Bible said of the children of Israel, "For the LORD your God is bringing you into a good land, a land of brooks of water, of fountains and springs, that flow out of valleys and hills; a land of wheat and barley, of vines and fig trees and pomegranates, a land of olive oil and honey" (Deuteronomy 8:7–8). This was the Promised Land, and it was described by what they would get to eat once they got there. God was saying, "Get ready! The food is going to be great, and you're going to love it. There's going to be lots of clean, fresh water. It's going to spring up from deep springs. It's going to flow down from the mountains. Make your kitchen into the Promised Land!"

"But I don't do vegetables, and very little fruit either," I hear you say. Well, that has to change. Remember that taste is acquired. There are places in the world where people eat grasshoppers and insect larvae. There are places where people eat animals we consider pets. *And they enjoy what they eat!* Taste is something we learn from our parents and our culture. Some of our learning has not been particularly good for our health. We have to unlearn the kinds of eating behavior that hurt us and relearn healthier ways of eating. You can learn to eat fruits and vegetables and enjoy them—and you must.

Okay, let's get into it and talk about what kinds of foods to eat. While this program doesn't try to tell you what you can eat and what you can't eat, there are some guidelines that will help you. First and foremost, shop for "live" foods. Live foods are those found around the outside aisles of the grocery store. That's where you find the fruits, vegetables, dairy products, meats, poultry, and fish that are so healthy for us. Down the inside aisles is where you find processed foods that are certainly not alive, and perhaps they have been on those shelves for months or years. Do you really want to focus on putting that kind of food—food often loaded with preservatives—into your body?

We can't say a lack of information is responsible for the overweight condition in which we, as a nation, find ourselves. The US Department of Agriculture (USDA) created an icon to help Americans make healthier food choices. The icon is shaped like a dinner plate in order to prompt people to think about building a healthy plate at mealtimes. At the USDA website (www.ChooseMyPlate.gov), you will see a plate icon that illustrates the five food groups using a place setting. At the website, you can also find more information and tips about making healthy food choices.

Registered dietitian Emily Ann Callahan, MPH, RD, states:

One thing that MyPlate reminds you to do is to make half of your plate fruits and vegetables. Almost any kind of fruit (fresh, frozen, canned, dried, or 100 percent fruit juice) is a good choice. A small amount of 100 percent fruit juice is okay and does provide some nutrients, but it does not provide the fiber that is necessary for good health the way that whole fruit does. Try to eat fruit in its whole state instead of drinking juice. When choosing canned fruit, look for fruits packed in 100 percent fruit juice or water instead of syrup, which has a lot of added sugar. Vegetables may be raw or cooked; fresh, frozen, canned, or dried/dehydrated. Choose a variety of colorful veggies; the USDA website has many ideas for including vegetables into your meals every day.

MyPlate shows that you should fill approximately one-quarter of your plate with grains. Any food made from wheat, rice, oats, cornmeal, barley, or another cereal grain is a grain product. Examples include bread, pasta, oatmeal, breakfast cereals, tortillas, and grits. Aim to choose whole grains for at least half of the grains you eat each day. Whole grains are made with the entire grain kernel and are more nutritious than refined grains such as white bread or white rice.

Proteins, which should take up approximately one-quarter of your plate, include meat, poultry, seafood, beans and peas, eggs, processed soy products, nuts, and seeds. Meat and poultry choices should be lean or low-fat. Look for leaner cuts of meat, such as sirloin or round steak. If meats are marbled with fat, they are not lean. Always trim off all visible fat. Seafood and plant proteins (soy, nuts, seeds, beans, and peas) are good protein alternatives to meat and poultry choices. Always bake, broil, or grill meat, poultry, and seafood instead of frying it, which adds a lot of calories and unhealthy fat.

Finally, the MyPlate icon includes the dairy group. All fluid milk products and many foods made from milk are considered part of this food group. Look for fat-free or low-fat dairy food choices, such as 1 percent or skim milk. Whole milk is not recommended for adults and children past the age of two years because of the unhealthy fat content. Dairy products are a great source of calcium, so if you don't drink milk or eat dairy products, you will need to look for other foods with high calcium content.[1]

The ChooseMyPlate website has many tools for helping you learn how to eat in a healthy manner. It's free, so use it to your health's advantage. Most of the information found there works well when you are at home. It's not too hard to keep track of what you are putting in your mouth when you are at home. Where you get into trouble is when you eat out. It used to be that Americans rarely ate out, but now most Americans eat out three or four times a week.

Learn to Read Labels

Learn to read nutrition labels on the back of food packages. You won't find nutrition labels on things like apples, apricots, and avocados, but they are on anything humans have processed. The government requires the food label to be there.

Ingredients List

Ingredients are listed in descending order by weight. The ingredient listed first is the heaviest, and the product is dominated by that ingredient. If any form of sugar is listed first, you should view that as a red flag. In the food products that are available today, there are many names and different forms of sugar, which I expand on in the section titled "Sugar" coming up.

Every food label also has a Daily Values column. While this is helpful information, remember that what you find there is a percentage of what you should have for the whole day and it is based on a 2,000-calorie-a-day diet.

Limit your intake not only of fat, but also of sodium (no more than 1,500 mg) and cholesterol. Pick those foods with high vitamin A and C. They are good choices. Look also for calcium and iron contents.

Calories per Serving

The first thing to look at when reading a label is the portion size. Many people don't consider this and think they are taking in fewer calories than they really are because instead of eating a half-cup serving of something, they have eaten a cup. A universal rule of thumb for weight loss is that if you burn 3,500 calories more than you take in, you will lose 1 pound. Therefore, if you reduce your intake by 500 calories per day, every day, you will lose 1 pound per week. And over the course of one year, that can add up to over 50 pounds lost. So what does 500 calories look like? A bagel with 3 ounces of cream cheese, a Venti Caramel Frappuccino at Starbucks, and two regular-size candy bars each contain about 500 calories.

Then check out the calories in a single serving. Calories are fuel for the body, and we need them to live, but if we have become overweight, it's an indication we have consistently taken in more calories than we can burn and the excess is being stored as fat. If you're going to lose weight, you are going to have to cut back on calories.

Sugar

Sugar is a hidden ingredient in many foods, and one for which you must carefully watch. When trying to identify sugar in food, look for both naturally occurring sugars and added sugars. Naturally occurring sugars are found in fruits and milk, while added sugars are those sugars that are added to foods. Look in the ingredients list for the following common names for the different forms of sugar: high fructose corn syrup or HFCS, sucrose, sucralose, fructose, dextrose, glucose, or other words ending in "-ose," corn syrup, fruit juice concentrate, honey, or maple syrup. These are just a few of the added sugars used in processed foods. In addition, you would be surprised by the food products that unexpectedly contain some form of sugar, including ketchup, salad dressing, barbeque sauce, tomato sauce, crackers, and some brands of peanut butter. When you are reading labels, it is best to avoid foods that have added sugars listed among the first few ingredients.

It is vitally important that you identify added sugars because not only do they contribute to obesity, but they also negatively affect your health. All forms of sugar you consume enter your intestinal tract, break down into glucose and fructose, and eventually reach your liver. An excess of sugar in the diet has been associated with very harmful fat buildup in the liver, which over a long period of time can lead to cirrhosis of the liver—not from alcohol but from sugar! Sugar is sugar. So watch for both types of sugar in foods, the naturally occurring kind and the added sugars in your favorite foods.

Fats

Next look at the fat grams. Fat is dense, and a little fat can pack a lot of calories. There are healthy fats and there are dangerous trans fats. Trans fat is the common name for a type of unsaturated fat with *trans*-isomer fatty acid. These fats can increase the risk of heart disease by raising LDL (bad cholesterol) and lowering HDL (good cholesterol).

Some people have tried to eliminate all fats from their diet. It's not a smart thing to do. Everyone needs some fat in their diet to maintain healthy cells, a strong nervous system, and good skin and hair. However, these fats should be mono-unsaturated fats such as those found in nuts, olive oil, and other unsaturated oils. Omega 3 oils, found in fish, nuts, and olive oil, for example, are necessary for good health.

Healthy fats are necessary for the ultimate functioning of the body and mind. They promote a healthy heart. They help prevent cancer. They keep down inflammation. They benefit nerve cells in the eyes and promote eye health. Because the brain is 60 percent fat, fat is necessary for healthy communication between the brain and nervous system. The right fats improve your mood and help in weight loss by increasing satisfaction from the foods you eat so that you will eat less. Unfortunately, the body does not differentiate between types of fats, and so all fats—good and bad—contribute to weight. We need healthy oils, but we need them in moderation.

Fiber

Check out the fiber grams on the label. You want to choose foods with a high fiber content, as most Americans don't eat enough fiber. You need 30 grams of fiber every day to keep the body functioning at its optimum. Here are some words of advice from Dr. Darren Baroni, board certified gastroenterologist:

> Eating fiber is very important to digestive tract health and general health overall. The more insoluble fiber that is in a person's diet, the less time bowel waste (and potential cancer causing substances called carcinogens) spend in the small intestine and colon. Fiber has been shown to be protective against colon cancer and probably against precancerous polyps. Additionally, fiber is more filling than other food ingredients and because, for the most part, it cannot be fully digested is lower in its overall caloric content. Hmmm, food

that fills you up but is not high in calories—doesn't that sound like a perfect food? This is not surprising given it comes from a perfect Creator! Foods high in fiber are whole grains, raw fruits, and most vegetables.[2]

Make wise choices with your food purchases. Read those labels and know what you are putting in your mouth. It matters. It makes a difference, and the difference shows up in added weight or loss of weight.

How Much Shall You Eat?

You need to eat enough to fuel your body so that it is at peak efficiency for what God wants you to do in life. God intended that you glorify Him with your body in your eating. First Corinthians 10:31 says, "Whether you eat or drink, or whatever you do, do all to the glory of God." Even your eating can glorify God. Maybe the last time you went to church you said, "I'm going to go worship and glorify God." That's wonderful! But in the same way, you can glorify Him when you go to lunch after church. I'll be honest: I'm not sure about all the ways you can glorify God by what you eat, but I am sure that overeating and gluttony are not among them (see Proverbs 23:1–3).

Some time ago, I was asked, "What would Jesus eat?" I thought about that question and decided He was probably not a vegetarian (see John 21:12–13; Luke 15:23). I don't think He would overeat, either. I think He would have eaten the diet of the culture, but in moderation. And we already know He exercised, because He walked everywhere He needed to go.

Water, Water, Water

Many people, like Carol, don't drink a lot of water. Rather, they drink sugar-loaded soft drinks. Carol was easily fatigued and she found that soft drinks with sugar made her feel better. It was addictive. She drank about four soft drinks a day to get a boost. She has since learned that not only do these sugared drinks cause one to be overweight, but they are also bad for your joints.

"I finally realized that all that sugar in the colas was affecting my weight. I stopped drinking them and looked for something to replace them," Carol said. "In the beginning, I drank fruit juices. Then I looked for something to drink that has protein. I began to drink Glucerna and other meal replacement drinks. The problem was that they too have lots of sugar. Then I began to drink a lot more water. It satisfied my cravings. Probably the biggest reason why I lost 15 pounds during my weight-loss competition was that I gave up drinking sugared colas."

Carol learned that water can be more satisfying than sugared soft drinks. Let's talk some more about water and its importance to life. Water is the most common and important liquid on Earth. Seventy percent of the earth's surface is covered with water. Life is impossible without it, and all known forms of life depend on it.

In the body, water works to transport nutrients and oxygen all through the body. It functions as a lubricant and a coolant. It is used for respiration, regulating the body's temperature, increasing metabolism, and is necessary for the removal of body wastes.

In addition, water maintains muscle tone, gives us clear and healthy skin, and, of course, assists in weight loss. It helps prevent lower back pain, chronic fatigue, headaches and migraines, asthma, allergies, arthritis, rheumatoid arthritis, hypertension, high cholesterol, muscle pain, neck pain, joint pain, constipation, ulcers, stomach pain, confusion and disorientation, and there is even some research that ties lack of water intake to Alzheimer's disease. More research with regard to the Alzheimer's connection is needed, but it is something to watch.

Water is a great aid in losing weight because it is calorie-free, has no fat or cholesterol, and is low in sodium. Water acts as an appetite suppressant, decreases fat deposits, increases muscle mass, keeps the kidneys functioning properly, and minimizes water retention.

Healthy kidneys can filter more than 500 ounces of water a day, but the highest recommended daily allowance in moderate climates is 129 ounces a day. Remember that only about 20 percent of your recommended daily allowance of water comes from other beverages and foods.

To help you increase your intake of water, start the day with a glass of water. Then throughout the day, don't wait until you are thirsty to drink. If you're thirsty, you are already dehydrated. Set a timer to remind you to drink water throughout the day. Add ice or lemon to your drink if you like. And choose vegetables every day that are high in water content.

What to Do When You Want to Cheat

The Bible tells us that the very first temptation ever was one involving food. Submitting to temptation with regard to food is as old as the Garden of Eden. "So when the woman saw that the tree was good for food, that it was pleasant to the eyes, and a tree desirable to make one wise, she took of its fruit and ate. She also gave to her husband with her, and he ate" (Genesis 3:6).

There it is. Eve looked, she saw, she desired it, she ate, and she gave it to Adam. We haven't progressed very far from that scenario. We look, we see, we want it, we eat it, and we may give it to someone else, causing him or her to give in to temptation as well. Eve's battle was to not eat the fruit; however, our battle is to eat fruit. Many of us don't like fruit, but that's because we've not made eating fruit a habit.

If we are overweight, we have a huge challenge. Because we are creatures of habit, our bodies resist change. And when we finally do make a change, our bodies want to revert to the old ways. I know this is true. I had a habit of eating ice cream every night for forty-eight years. I probably didn't go to bed more than ten times without eating ice cream. I had a deeply ingrained habit that was hard for me to break. Here's what I did.

When I started Bod4God, I had a cheat *meal*. Not a cheat day or week—a cheat meal on Friday night. Just one meal. When I had a craving—maybe on Tuesday—I postponed that craving to eat at my cheat meal on Friday night. I looked forward to that time when I could have the pizza I had been craving all week. The cheat meal was a big help to me in retraining my eating habits. I don't need a cheat meal now because I've changed. You may be trying hard to change, but you're not there yet, and so you need a cheat meal.

You have to bring your body into subjection. You can do this. Did you know that taste is developed? It is a learned behavior. You might not have a taste for healthy food, but you *can* change that. In Mark 1:6, we learn that John the Baptist ate locusts and wild honey. How would you like a nice plate of locusts with honey drizzled all over it. It looks gross to me, but if John were here, he probably wouldn't want a quarter pounder with cheese or Breyer's ice cream. He would prefer his locusts and honey because that's what he learned to like.

It's time to tell your body what it's going to do rather than letting it tell you what it wants. You might not like water, but if you keep drinking your full quota of water every day, you will develop a taste for it. Claim the promises found in 1 Corinthians 10:13, which says, "No temptation has overtaken you except such as is common to man; but God is faithful, who will not allow you to be tempted beyond what you are able, but with the temptation will also make the way of escape, that you may be able to bear it." Will you choose to take the way of escape?

Three Things to Do When You Want to Cheat

1. Pray Consistently

You have to understand that part of overcoming temptation involves prayer. Luke 18:1 says, "Men always ought to pray, and not lose heart." Your choices are to pray and be victorious, or not pray and faint. Pray about your exercise. Pray about your eating habits. Tell God that you've stopped looking for the quick fix—the magic pill—and you are ready to let Him help you. He will.

Be proactive and pray positively for healthy habits and not just negatively for your health problems. When I ask people what their prayer needs are, often what I hear in response is an "organ recital." You know, "I have a weak kidney," or, "I have diabetes," or, "The doctor is worried about my heart." It would be so exciting to hear, "Pastor, pray for me to drink more water." That would be a positive, preventive prayer of faith.

2. Shop Carefully

The rule of thumb is this: if food gets near you, it will eventually get in you. The battleground is not your kitchen—it's the grocery store. Shop for your health, not your happiness. If you keep what you shouldn't eat out of your basket, you'll keep it out of your car; and if you keep it out of the car, you'll keep it out of your house. I've literally stood at the checkout counter and thought, *What am I doing with this food?* I've put it back rather than take it to the car and home. In Romans 13:14, Paul says, "Put on the Lord Jesus Christ, and make no provision for the flesh, to fulfill its lusts." Here are some tips for healthy grocery shopping:

- Don't go shopping when you are hungry. The temptation may just be too great.

- Pray for the filling of the Holy Spirit before you go into the store. I pray, "Oh God, fill me right now." I don't want to fulfill the lust of my flesh.

- Remember to shop on the outside aisles of the store where the living food is.

- Take the time to read the labels. Know what's in the food that you eat.

- Purchase some healthy snacks. I like fruit and almonds. Almonds are a plant-based protein high in fiber. They are filling and satisfying and help to promote good heart health. I eat a handful every day.

3. Think Correctly

In 2 Corinthians 10:4–5, Paul says, "The weapons of our warfare are not carnal, but mighty through God to the pulling down of strong holds; casting down imaginations, and every high thing that exalteth itself against the knowledge of God, and bringing into captivity every thought to the obedience of Christ" (KJV). In this case, and for us, "imaginations" are food cravings. What happens is that we start thinking about our cravings. If we don't cast down our imaginations—clear out our minds and let the Holy Spirit take control—we will give in to our cravings. Remember that every sin begins in the mind. We can't afford to let sinful thoughts stay in our minds.

There is a kind of detrimental thinking I call "Esau thinking." In Genesis 25, we find the story of Esau, who had been out hunting all day. He came to Jacob and said, "Please feed me with that same red stew, for I am weary." Jacob took advantage of the situation and replied, "Sell me your birthright." In that culture, the elder son took precedence over his younger brother. After the father's death, he would acquire a double portion of inheritance. Esau ignored all of that and said, "Look, I am about to die; so what is this birthright to me?" He sold it right then and there.

The Bible doesn't let it go. Hebrews 12:16 calls Esau a profane person who sold his birthright for one morsel of meat. Esau could have had so much, but he gave it all up for a dish of soup. He thought he had to have short-term pleasure and that it was worth more than his inheritance. What about your health? You know that some of the stuff you put in your mouth is not good for you. You know it and yet you do it.

Instead of "Esau thinking," we need to have "Moses thinking." Moses's parents feared God more than they feared Pharaoh. They hid him until they just couldn't hide him any longer. Later, when Moses came of age, he refused to live in Pharaoh's house. To Moses, short-term pleasure was not worth the long-term pain of seeing his people suffer. Don't be fooled. Sin is fun—for a season. Moses made the choice (see Hebrews 11:24–27). He walked away from everything because he had right thinking. In the midst of plenty such as we have in this country, you have to remember that long-term health is not worth the short-term pleasure of junk food.

My friends, failure is not final. If you cheat—learn from it. Get back on track right away. The Bible says, "For a righteous man may fall seven times and rise again" (Proverbs 24:16). Ninety percent of life is just showing up. You've showed up. You're here. Keep showing up. Keep taking those small steps to health.

A Bod4God Close-Up

Bad News Turned Around

Arlene Spann
Lost 50 pounds

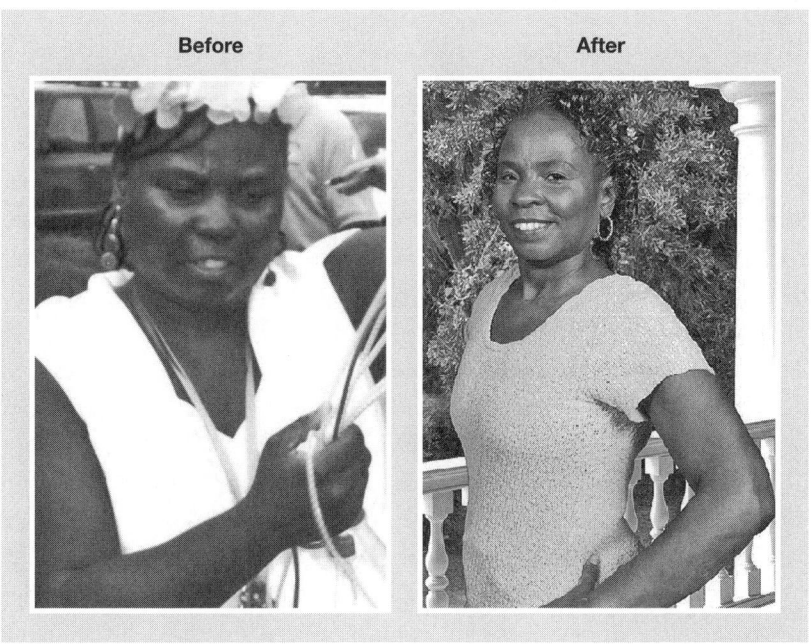

Before   After

"I've got good news, and I've got bad news." Don't you hold your breath just a little bit when you hear those words? Well . . . I have good news and bad news for you. The good news is that Jesus came to give us life, and life more abundant. The bad news is that there is a thief, Satan, who comes to steal, kill, and destroy us. I got angry when I realized he was trying to destroy me through my bad health choices.

I had no idea that my health was at risk until my doctor said, "You are overweight." I had weighed around 125 pounds most of my young adult life. However, I experienced several deaths of people in my life, and the inability to grieve and other life challenges had caused my weight to sky-rocket to an unhealthy 183 pounds. It was that doctor's visit that started me on my weight-loss journey. During that visit, I learned that I had high cholesterol, was pre-diabetic, and was overweight. I knew what it meant to have diabetes. My mother, my grandmother, and my aunt were all diabetic, so I knew the seriousness of what my doctor was telling me. Pills were not an option for me, so I asked my doctor what I could do. She said that I could start watching what I ate to see if that would help get my blood sugar under control.

But even after receiving this shocking news, I did not begin immediately. I just couldn't motivate myself. I tried a few things like walking and exercising a little, but I found it hard to continue alone. Then I learned about the Losing To Live program at my church, Woodstream Church in Upper Marlboro, Maryland, and I was moved to sign up. God began to renew my thinking because of the Bible-centered keys to weight loss: dedication, inspiration, eat, exercise, and team. I have been able to shed nearly 50 pounds by being a part of the Losing To Live Weight-Loss Program. I also discovered healthier eating habits like eliminating soft drinks and processed foods and how to use spices instead of adding salt to foods. I learned about drinking more water and using healthier sweeteners like Stevia.

After learning that Christians are statistically the most overweight group of people, I began to see why we should be concerned about our health. We are God's representatives, and we should honor Him with our bodies. As Christians, we should come to realize that we are not our own. Our bodies are to be dedicated to God for His use. I have learned through memorizing Galatians 5:16, which says, "Walk in the Spirit, and you shall not fulfill the lust of the flesh," that we need the Holy Spirit to help us control the flesh. My biggest struggle to this day is the temptation to revert back and eat unhealthy foods. However, I am determined to live a healthy life and to keep my blood sugar under control. A big motivation for me is that I do not want to be forced to give myself insulin like other family members have had to do.

In order to keep on track, I made several changes to my eating habits. The first thing I did was drink more water. This is so important. I also cut out fried foods and replaced them with baked foods, I cut back on snack foods like chips and candy, and I ate more greens. I even began to eat more raw vegetables and fruits. For exercise, I began to walk and move more. I danced, mopped, ran, did jumping jacks, did push-ups, and got on the elliptical machine. I even took Pastor Steve's advice and parked farther away from the entrance at church and at stores. I learned through the program that God wants us to move. So I did. Just recently I completed my first 5K race. It was such an accomplishment for me, one I will never forget.

I want to encourage you to let others help you along your journey to a healthier life. My Losing To Live team has helped me so much by being competitive, motivating, and holding me accountable. They also gave me a sense that I was not on this journey alone. It was wonderful having others to celebrate with and keep me accountable for what I consumed during the week and what I did for exercise. My leader helped me see certain Scripture verses in a different light. It was as if a lightbulb went off in my mind when reading God's Word. I was now associating certain passages with how they related to my body. She asked me the tough questions like whether or not my eating habits were based on emotion. She also taught me so many practical tips, such as how to read labels and the dangers of high fructose corn syrup. In fact, my team leader had such an influence on me and my success that I am now committed to do the same for others and am currently a team leader in the program.

I love to show people a pair of my favorite pants from before I lost all my weight. They are a size 16, and I remember how I thought I looked fit and good in them. I am now a size 6, 10 sizes smaller! I attribute this transformation to the Losing To Live program and the principles I learned in it. I no longer have to get shots for my tennis elbow, no longer suffer from swollen joints, and no longer have the aches and pains that I once suffered with. And praise God, I am now free from the threat of diabetes! When I embraced what God was saying to me through His Word about my health and body, my life really changed. The Lord wants us to be in good health. I know that I still have a lot more work to do, and I know that the Lord is not through with me yet. Remember, you are a part of God's body, so let's be the best representatives of Him that we can. Losing To Live is for a lifetime. This program truly saved my life!

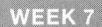

Small Steps to Life Ideas

Have you weighed in? How are you doing? If you have been faithful to the small steps to life, you have probably lost some weight—maybe even a lot of weight.

What Do You Need to Know about H_2O?

This chapter has a lot more good information about water. Don't neglect to drink an adequate amount of water every day. Let's stop and thank God for water. "Thank You, God, for rain and ice and snow. Bless you, Father, for being Jehovah Jirah, the God who provides water so we can drink what we need and take care of our bodies. Amen."

Small Food Step

Plan your snacks. Successful dieters eat about six small meals a day to maintain their metabolism. Eating small meals like this keeps a steady flow of glucose to the body. Here are some ideas for eating more healthy snacks:

- Spread a tablespoon of peanut butter on apple slices.
- Toss dried cranberries and chopped nuts—walnuts or almonds—in a bowl of instant oatmeal.
- Top fat-free or low-fat vanilla yogurt with crunchy granola—a tablespoon or two—and add blueberries.
- Have fat-reduced microwave popcorn and sprinkle it with a bit of Parmesan cheese for flavor, but do not add butter or margarine.
- Put nonfat frozen whipped topping between two graham or chocolate graham crackers for an "ice-cream sandwich."
- Dip bits and pieces of veggies in nonfat dressing.
- Dip strawberries or apple slices in nonfat yogurt.

Small Exercise Step

Learn some exercises you can do at your desk or while traveling in a car or airplane. Do some leg lifts by lifting your feet off the ground and holding them up for a few seconds while tightening your abs. Do this several times a day for several weeks and you will begin to have tighter abs. Remember that muscle burns fat even when your body is at rest.

Bod4God Victory Guide

Remember that *the victory is in the Victory Guide*. Record your progress on My Progress Report located on page 22.

Week 7: *E* Is for Eat

Bod4God Thought

Eat for your health, not your happiness.

Bod4God Memory Verse

Each of you should know how to possess his own vessel in sanctification and honor. (1 Thessalonians 4:4)

Bod4God Reflection/Application Questions

1. What does Paul mean in 1 Thessalonians 4:4 when he writes, "Each of you should know how to possess his own vessel"?

   ....

   ....

   ....

   ....

   ....

2. What is the connection between obedience to God and managing your eating habits?

   ....

   ....

   ....

   ....

   ....

3. We often find ways to abuse God's perfect gifts, such as food. In what ways have you abused God's gift of food?

....

....

....

....

....

4. In what ways are you using food to meet needs other than nourishment in your life?

....

....

....

....

....

5. Gluttony is an action that reflects a person who is controlled by appetite. When are you most vulnerable to gluttony?

....

....

....

....

....

6. What foods tempt you the most?

....

....

....

....

....

7. What steps do you need to take to make sure you are consuming enough water each day?

....

....

....

....

....

8. After reading this chapter's Bod4God Close-Up, what can you relate to and what can you take from this person's story to apply to your own life and lifestyle plan?

....

....

....

....

....

Bod4God Small Steps to Life Record

What "Skinny Things" Will You Do This Week?

Fill out this chart by indicating: (1) what you will do to eat less to live; (2) what you will do to exercise more to live; and (3) how many average daily ounces of water you will drink. Pick only a few things, and stick with them. Remember that weight loss and maintenance require you to *eat less* and *exercise more*.

Sun.	
Mon.	
Tues.	
Wed.	
Thurs.	
Fri.	
Sat.	

My Bod4God Journal

Teach me, O Lᴏʀᴅ, the way of Your statutes, and I shall keep it to the end.

Psalm 119:33

Record what God is telling you to do this week to apply the four keys to lasting weight loss.

Dedication: Honoring God with My Body

....

....

....

....

Inspiration: Motivating Myself for Change

....

....

....

....

Eat and Exercise: Managing My Habits

....

....

....

....

Team: Building My Circle of Support

....

....

....

....

....

E Is for Exercise

It Is Better to Exercise an Hour a Day than to Be Dead Twenty-four Hours a Day

> Therefore, whether you eat or drink, or whatever you do, do all to the glory of God.
>
> 1 Corinthians 10:31

Do you have to exercise for the rest of your life? Yes, you do. There is no way around the fact that permanent weight loss comes only to those who exercise. Read any of the stories in this book and you will see that eating less and exercising more are the keys to health and a trim body. Exercise in *Bod4God* simply means moving your body. Every time you move your body you exercise. That doesn't mean you have to join a body builders class or spend all day at the gym. There are small steps to life you can do that begin to benefit your body right away. What's encouraging is that all of the people in our stories began to feel better when they shed a few pounds and got moving. But let's face it, people who are overweight have difficulty exercising. However, the more you move, the more you lose, and the more you lose, the more you want to move. It's so simple, but so true.

When Did Exercise Become a Problem?

God made us to be physically active. When God created man, as recorded in Genesis 2, He put him in a garden and said, "Get to work. Tend the garden." If you've ever done extensive gardening, you know that it exercises every muscle in your body. I'm sure that there were vines to be cut back, crops to be harvested, and perhaps even seeds to be planted.

Then, when Adam and Eve sinned and were driven from the Garden of Eden, their work *truly* began. Now they had to fight the earth. God said, "In the sweat of your face you shall eat bread" (Genesis 3:19). Things were not going to come easily to this couple anymore, and things don't come easily to us either. We have to work for what we get.

God intended for us to be physically active. In the last one hundred years, things have changed. We have gone from being an agrarian society to being a technological society. We've gone from fifteen-hour days in the field to fifteen-hour days in front of a computer screen. We've gone from being physically active to being physically inactive. And it hasn't done our society any good. The sedentary lifestyle most of us now follow has contributed to the problem of obesity in this country. And in recent years, it has been getting worse. A recent study published by the Washington University School of Medicine determined that obese Americans now outnumber those who are merely overweight. As of 2012, 67.6 million Americans were classified as obese, while an additional 65.2 million were classified as overweight.[1] This is an alarming trend.

There is nothing wrong with doing sedentary work as long as you realize you have to compensate for the lack of exercise in your line of work by being intentional about exercise. You have to schedule exercise into your life or it won't happen. I'm sure your head is nodding as you read this. You know what I mean, don't you?

There is only one Scripture passage in the Bible that mentions the word *exercise*. It is found in 1 Timothy 4:8, where Paul writes to Timothy, "For bodily exercise profits a little." I loved this verse, and if anybody talked about exercise, I would remind those people that it profited only "a little." However, that verse is a comparative statement. It is comparing physical exercise to spiritual exercise. When we exercise physically, we are taking care of the temporal. When we exercise spiritually, we're taking care of the eternal.

Some of you are out of balance in this area. Some of you are physically active and in perfect shape, but you never read your Bible, pray, or go to church as you should. You have abs and biceps to prove that you are strong physically, but you don't have the spiritual muscles you need to survive in this world. You need to exercise spiritually. All of us will die one day, and we'd better be investing ourselves in something that's going to outlast us, something of eternal significance. That's what the Timothy verse is teaching us. We can't use that verse as an excuse not to exercise, because God has told us to be physically active. We have to become more intentional about getting enough exercise.

By the way, look again at that verse in 1 Timothy. Paul doesn't say that exercise profits us nothing. He says it does profit us, but only a little compared to the pursuit of spiritual strength. We need both physical exercise and spiritual exercise. The Olympic Games began hundreds of years before Paul wrote those words in his letter to Timothy. The Romans and the Greeks were seriously into games in which physical strength and endurance were essential, and lack of strength and endurance often cost players their lives. But what was the *spiritual* strength of these athletes? In many cases, it was probably nonexistent. The players were probably worshipers of both the gods and the emperor.

So if you are one of those people who has a great physique, but you never look between the covers of your Bible and you never pray, remember that bodily exercise profits only "a little."

What Are the Benefits of Exercise?

The benefits of exercise are multiple. Exercise helps your body in almost every conceivable way. One of the greatest benefits of exercise is that it helps you lose weight. Only a small percentage of people can lose weight without exercise, but 100 percent of people have to exercise to be healthy. Remember that in the time of the Bible, people had no cars. They walked with seemingly little regard for distance. While not having transportation may seem like a problem, for these people it was a blessing in disguise. They didn't have to go to the gym every day. They got plenty of exercise. On the other hand, we don't walk everywhere like that and we have to make sure that we are exercising enough to gain benefits from it.

The most important step in establishing a fitness program is to do *something*. You can choose any kind of exercise that works for you. You can do cardio or strength and flexibility programs. You can decide if you want to work out with a group or do it alone. Many people exercise alone, but there is nothing like working out and exercising with a buddy to keep you on task and accountable.

Ask yourself the question, "What sabotages my attempts to exercise?" Make whatever that thing is a matter of prayer and planning.

You need to start exercising slowly. If you go all out on your first day and then become so sore you can't exercise again the next day, you haven't gained much. Remember, this is a lifestyle change, and real change can come slowly. Make sure you stretch before exercising to prevent injury and soreness. Keep track of how often you exercise. Keep your exercise routine simple. It might help to play music, perhaps praise songs, while you exercise. Maybe you can listen to an audiobook or podcast on your smartphone or do your Scripture memory work while you are exercising. Vary your workout to use all seven muscle groups. This is called cross-training.

Exercise must become a habit—a sacred appointment you keep with God and yourself. God designed us to function best when we move our bodies. We were not fashioned to live sedentary lives filled with stress. So choose an active lifestyle.

How Much Exercise Is Enough?

If you have to ask that question, you are probably not getting enough exercise. The US Surgeon General recommends that adults engage in at least 150 minutes of moderate-intensity physical activity each week, and supplement aerobic activities with muscle-training activities that involve all muscle groups at least two days a week.[2] As always, check with your health care provider and a fitness professional for personalized exercise recommendations.

Exercise books are a dime a dozen in secondhand shops, and they all say pretty much the same thing. So if you are strapped for cash, use your money to get a good pair of athletic shoes and pick up a secondhand book on exercise. You don't need a fancy gym membership, although many people enjoy the camaraderie they find in exercising with other folks. An exercise pal is a good thing to have; you can encourage each other to get going on days when one or the other doesn't feel like moving.

Our church partners with a ministry called Body & Soul: Where Faith and Fitness Meet (www.bodyandsoul.org) to offer an awesome exercise program that provides cardio and strength training fitness set to contemporary Christian music. Body & Soul was developed by fitness specialists Jeannie and Roy Blocher in Germantown, Maryland.

This ministry equips fitness-minded Christians to lead exercise classes both in the church and in the community. They also provide an encouraging environment for Christians to improve their health and invite their non-Christian friends to do the same. Jeannie Blocher says, "Develop an exercise program that motivates you to do it day after day. You want to wake up each day saying about your exercise program, 'I can do that again today.' The most important thing about exercise is not what you do but that you do it." Here are some of Jeannie's ideas:

- If you love the outdoors, walk, jog, bike, hike, or skate.
- If you want to pamper your joints and like the water, swim.
- Use a rocking chair instead of a regular chair.
- Find something you like to do that involves repetitious movement.
- Breathe deeply and forcefully several times a day to aerate your entire lungs.
- Go dancing, particularly square dancing, for fun and good exercise for all ages.
- Try a group fitness class, especially a faith-based one that offers a safe, caring environment, whether you are a beginner or a veteran exerciser.
- If you like competition, go for team sports—basketball, soccer, or local softball teams.
- Have a family meeting where you decide how each member is going to participate in fitness.
- Plant the value of fitness in your kids at an early age and it will always be part of their lifestyle.
- Plan active vacations in which you build some time around physical activity. [3]

The One Exercise That Fits All

Perhaps one of the easiest and best ways to get the exercise you need is to walk. The old Nike ad said it so clearly—"Just do it!" Just put on your shoes and get walking. Walking has so many benefits in addition to exercise. If you are having a relationship problem with someone, take a walk with him or her. It's a great opportunity to begin communication. Walking is a great time to pray. It's a great time to get out and enjoy nature.

Walking Clubs

Jesus walked with His disciples. Why not join a walking club and enjoy short walks and long hikes? A walking club will provide safety for members, and encouragement from other walkers will help you to keep exercising.

Our church has a walking club we call the 100-Mile Club. The goal is for participants to walk at least 100 miles over a twelve-week period. We meet every Sunday evening for twelve weeks for a group walk. That gives a physical affirmation of our commitment to God, our bodies, our families, and the Losing To Live fellowship.

We meet at the church to start our walk, and we walk the 5K route we will use for that event. We modify the course into A, B, and C courses, depending on the walker's fitness level. The course is beautiful and God-inspired.

Mall Walking

Another walking option is mall walking. Many malls open their doors as early as 6:00 a.m. for people who want to use their facilities for exercise. People who walk in malls quickly get acquainted with each other and often form friendships. Usually, a regular walker will know how many laps of the mall you must take to walk a mile. You can walk early in the morning, any time during the day, or in the early evening. But remember that there are peak times when the malls are crowded, and if you walk during those times, you will be constantly swerving to avoid shoppers. Mall walking provides shelter during rainy or wintry days, so there's no excuse not to walk!

Count Your Steps

If you are walking alone, a good way to motivate yourself is to get a device that counts your steps and use it every day. The goal should be 10,000 steps a day. It will take a while to build up to that number of steps, but it won't happen if you don't start.

Go to a high-end sporting goods store and invest in a good pedometer. Bad pedometers will only frustrate and discourage you, as they do not accurately record your distance. (You can do online research for the various brands of pedometers available by typing "pedometer reviews" into a search engine.)

There are also a variety of apps and fitness trackers that can help you track your steps. Research the different ways to keep track of your 10,000 steps and find the tool that works best for you and your lifestyle.

Shoes

Walking shoes are your most important item of gear, so plan to buy the best pair you can afford. You are worth the price. There is not a "best" shoe for everyone. The best shoe for you is the one that fits your foot and activity. If you've wondered whether to buy running shoes or walking shoes, buy the running shoes. That's because shoe manufacturers put their design resources into running shoes. Walking shoes are often little more than "pretty shoes."

If you start to take walking seriously and decide to walk in the mountains or go on a walking trip in this country or abroad, you might want to wear boots. While boots are inflexible and heavy, they are great for walking on uneven surfaces such as you might find on a trail or on cobblestones in Europe. Boots also protect the ankles from being turned and sprained.

Shop for shoes in the morning so that your feet will not be swollen. Take your time when buying walking shoes. Put on the shoes—both of them—and walk around the store for a while. Fitting problems should show up before you leave the store. When you get home, wear the shoes indoors for a few days in case you need to return them to the store.

Keep track of how many miles you have put on your shoes. They should be replaced before they have 600 miles on them because they lose their support. If you are overweight, you are hard on your shoes, or the shoes are lightweight, you may need to replace them closer to 300 miles. This is important, so even if your shoes don't look worn out, replace them anyway.

A good pair of walking shoes will probably cost $75 to $150. Remember, you are worth it and you can use the money you save because you're not buying a lot of expensive junk food.

What Are Some Other Ways to Exercise?

Do a few stretches early in the morning to get your metabolism started. Dance around while you brush your teeth. Do heel lifts while the coffee is brewing. Our Losing To Live participants find ways to exercise that fit their unique lifestyles and schedules. Some people swim or work out at a gym facility. Sabrina Prime, a wife and mom who has lost over 80 pounds, joined a gym using a ninety-day free offer coupon. She made such good use of the gym's offerings that she decided to rejoin when the ninety days were up.

Some participants get out and walk before breakfast. Some wait until just after breakfast. Some walk at noon when the day is the warmest. Some walk in the evening after work to get rid of tension. You have to find your own routine and stick to it.

Check off the small actions listed below that you can do right away to get started exercising and then make them part of your daily life just like brushing your teeth or combing your hair. The most important thing is that you take your exercise just as you would take a prescription:

- Do it three to five times a week—regularly.
- Pick a partner or exercise buddy to stay motivated.
- Plan ahead and set aside a regular exercise time.
- Keep track of your exercise program and be proud of yourself every day that you do it.
- Update your friends and family on your successes.
- Train, don't strain. Start slowly and gradually build up.
- Watch your diet and eat wisely.

A great website with video demonstrations of various exercises and other recommendations to get you started *and* to keep you motivated is that of the Centers for Disease Control (CDC): http://www.cdc.gov/physical activity/everyone/videos/.

Setting Exercise Goals

You need two kinds of goals: goals of output and goals of input. Let me explain. I set out to lose 100 pounds. That was my goal of output. But to reach that goal, I had to have goals of input. I had to drink the water I was supposed to drink. I had to exercise at least three times a week. I had to eat properly. These were my goals of input. So, too, must you establish goals of input to achieve your output goal.

Additionally, it helps to recognize that your output goal is a statement of faith in God's ability to help you achieve it. When you state your goal, say it in faith. "I will lose 30 pounds by Thanksgiving." Jesus said about faith that we are to say to the mountain, "Be removed" (Matthew 21:21). You have to have faith that you will have a healthier future. You are painting a vision of what you want your life to look like.

In Habakkuk 2:2, God instructed the prophet, "Write the vision and make it plain on tablets, that he may run who reads it." Can I remind you again to write down your exercise goal and put it where you can see it? Keep your goal in front of you.

Now, let's talk for a moment about goal setting.

1. An exercise goal must be *specific*. "I want to walk" isn't a specific goal. But if you say, "I will walk 30 minutes every day," that's a specific goal. At first, maybe you can't walk for 30 minutes at one time. Set some intermittent goals that will get you to that 30-minute goal. You also have to strive to reach at least a moderately brisk pace.

2. An exercise goal must be *achievable*. The average person is going to lose about 1 to 2 pounds a week. If you are extremely heavy, as I was, you may lose weight faster than that. In order to accelerate the weight loss, you have to exercise. In the beginning, set an achievable exercise goal.

3. The exercise goal must be *measurable*. That's the easy part. All you have to do is stand on a scale to see if you are reaching your weight goal. An exercise goal can be measured by using a pedometer or staking out a route of, say, 1 mile. Drive it in your car to measure the distance, then park the car and get walking.

If you are faithful in walking and eating healthy foods in small portions, you will lose weight. Then, stepping on the scale becomes a joyful experience as your weight creeps slowly downward.

A group of doctors who studied obese and overweight adults found that those who weighed themselves more often lost more weight and prevented more weight gain over a period of two years than those who weighed themselves less frequently. Contrary to the advice given in many popular weight-loss regimens, this study suggests that at least some people can benefit from the accountability brought on by daily weigh-ins. Potential advantages of daily weighing include the recognition of slow patterns of weight gain that may not be immediately apparent and the chance to modify lifestyle habits before the total weight gain becomes extreme and difficult to control.

One caveat: because your weight fluctuates from day to day, daily weighing can lead to discouragement and potential diet sabotage if you see a higher number from one day to the next. Most diet experts believe that a weekly or even a monthly weigh-in is a more accurate reflection of weight-loss progress. I prefer the once-a-week weigh-in.

Your personality will likely play a role in deciding how often to weigh yourself. If you're easily discouraged, daily weighing might cause you to give up your attempts if you don't see rapid progress. On the other hand, if you crave control and feedback, daily weighing might satisfy more of your needs and fuel your motivation. Whatever weigh-in frequency you choose, keep these tips in mind when stepping on the scale:

1. Weighing yourself first thing in the morning is usually best. Because of variations in food and fluid consumption, we often "gain" different amounts of weight throughout the day.

2. If you're weighing frequently, remember that daily fluctuations in weight are common. Just because you're heavier today than yesterday doesn't mean your weight-loss program isn't working. Don't become a slave to the numbers.

3. Monthly variations in weight are also common in menstruating women.

4. Plateaus in weight loss aren't necessarily bad. If you're exercising a lot, your weight may remain constant for a time as you build

muscle, even though you're still decreasing your body fat content and getting healthier.

5. Finally, cues other than the numbers on the scale are equally important. How do you feel? Are your clothes getting looser or tighter? Do you feel stronger, healthier, leaner? Your own perceptions can be the most valuable tool to help you track your weight-loss progress.

Getting your eating and exercising plans written down and under control is vital to achieving lasting weight loss. Try some of the tips you have read in the last few chapters and see what works for you. Remember, there are no magic pills or potions that will erase the years of neglect you have inflicted on your body. It takes a lot of hard work and determination to lose weight and keep it off. But you can do it. Start managing your eating and exercising habits, and you will see results. Now it's time to talk about joining a team of losers to help you succeed and achieve your weight-loss goals.

A Bod4God Close-Up

Fifty, Fit, and Fabulous

Lisa Nowalski
Lost 145 pounds

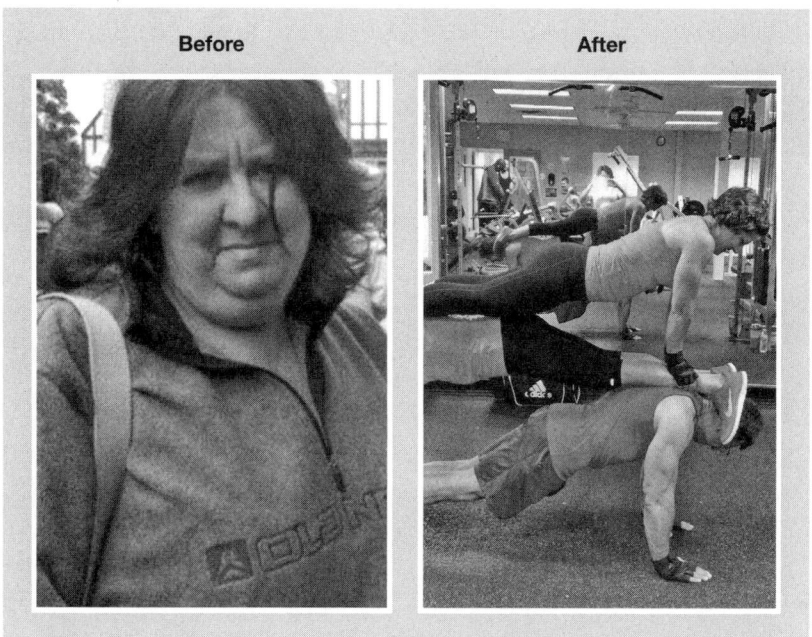

My transformation began with a 6-mile bike ride to the pharmacy to fill prescriptions. I weighed around 285 pounds, and my health was out of control. I was taking medications for high blood pressure, high cholesterol, chronic pain, depression, and migraines. I had struggled with my weight for most of my adult life. I knew I needed to change, but I just couldn't seem to do it. A defining moment in my life happened about twelve years ago when I was standing by my father's deathbed. I clearly remember him taking off his oxygen mask and telling me that if I didn't want to die like him, I needed to do something about the way I was living. Even though that statement felt like a slap in the face, I still could not seem to get motivated to change. I finally made the decision to change after I heard my pastor, Jamey Stewart of Believers Church in Chesapeake, Virginia, preach the Bod4God sermon series. I was ready. I knew I could not live like this any longer.

For a woman, starting to lose weight at the age of forty-seven can be an intimidating process. But I walked through the doors of the Taylor Bend Family YMCA in Chesapeake, Virginia, the day after that bike ride determined to achieve success. I went every day, and I listened to and took the advice of the trainers. I removed old unhealthy habits from my life and replaced them with healthy ones. I also followed what Pastor Jamey preached on honoring God with my body. My dedication, determination, and hard work paid off. I started my journey weighing in at 285 pounds. Now I weigh 140 pounds, have actual muscle mass, and am in the best shape of my life. I have developed a love for physical fitness and now enjoy exercising and lifting weights. Through the principles that I learned from Bod4God, I have been able to maintain this weight loss.

One of the small steps that I made to help jump-start my weight loss was removing the junk food from my house and replacing it with healthier food. This was very hard for me. To be honest, I cried. I acted like a two-year-old, throwing a temper tantrum on my living room floor. But I'm glad I did it. Cutting out junk food helped me shed the pounds. I had a previous operation on my back that caused problems with my feet and the way I walked. It was embarrassing for me, but I had to have my twenty-year-old daughter teach me how to walk on a treadmill. Even though I faced these obstacles, I was determined to get healthy, and I did not let anything slow me down. I began to love my cycling/spin class, and soon after that I began weight training.

I was recently admitted to the hospital with a serious case of ulcerative colitis. My doctor told me that if I wasn't in the shape I was in I would not have lived through the illness. I was in Intensive Care Unit for four days and in ICU stepdown for another four and a half weeks. I am still dealing with some residual health issues from it, but I still go to the gym daily and lift weights. I shudder when I think about what could have happened to me if I hadn't been in good physical condition before I became ill.

I so enjoy my time at the YMCA, and now I am able to work there. I currently teach a class that I once took called Y-Change, which teaches about nutrition and exercise. I also love that it is a Christian environment, and I am able to talk about what Christ has done in my life and hopefully inspire others through my story. It is so important for Christians to understand that the Holy Spirit lives within us. That is one of my biggest motivations in staying healthy.

Today, I live for Christ, and I am so thankful for His help in getting healthy. I struggle with being patient with others, and sometimes I have trouble realizing that everybody has a different starting point and different priorities when it comes to their health. I know that He is using me to help inspire people to get healthy and live their lives for Him. My Losing To Live team helped me stay on track by keeping me accountable. Publicly sharing my story on Facebook, with my church family, and with the members of the YMCA helped me stay focused. My friends would encourage me and compliment me on every pound I lost. I posted my weight and every time I walked into the gym not to draw attention to myself but rather to Jesus Christ and what He was doing in my life.

I never dreamed that I would be teaching health and fitness classes and helping others realize their responsibility in taking care of their temple, the residence of the Holy Spirit. I can honestly say that there is no better feeling than to see somebody get healthy, lose weight, and live for Jesus Christ. My advice to you is to get yourself in a good Bible-believing church so that you can get the help and accountability you need to succeed. I also strongly recommend joining a YMCA. They are affordable, and you are able to pray and speak about Jesus Christ openly.

Remember that bike ride to the pharmacy to buy all those medications? I am proud to share with you that I am now drug free, pain free, and migraine free. What a transformation! Shedding all of that weight took so much pressure off my body and enabled me to not be dependent on all the medications. But my story is not about me. It's about Jesus and what He can do for you and through you for His kingdom.

Small Steps to Life Ideas

What Do You Need to Know about H₂O?

Drinking a pint of water will increase metabolism for about half an hour, causing the body to burn about 25 calories. Researchers believe that the increase in metabolism comes from warming the water in the stomach. That means that if you drink a pint of water before a meal, you will rev up your metabolism as well as make your stomach feel full. It will help you eat less and burn more when you do eat your meal. Let's look at a couple more changes you can make in eating and exercise.

Small Food Step

How about a great recipe to encourage your healthy eating? This one is a healthy wrap. Wraps are great because they are creative, individual and versatile. For a great wrap, create a combination of the following ingredients:

1. Tortillas (whole wheat, tomato, spinach, roasted garlic)
2. Lean meat (turkey, roast beef, roasted chicken, grilled chicken, tuna, spicy shrimp, even leftover steak)
3. Salad greens or vegetables (lettuce, olives, salsa)
4. Low-fat cheese (cheddar, jalapeño jack, provolone)
5. Low-fat dressing (ranch, chipotle ranch, blue cheese, balsamic vinaigrette)

Spread salad dressing on the tortilla. (You might want to steam, microwave, or heat the tortilla so that it becomes soft for easy rolling.) Layer lean meat, cheese, and vegetables on the tortilla and then roll tightly. Cut and serve with a low-fat side dish (vinegar slaw, roasted vegetable salad, or a low-fat grain salad).

Small Exercise Steps

There are a number of small exercise steps given in this chapter already, but let's add one more: leg lifts while sitting at the computer. Do five reps, two to three times a day.

Bod4God Victory Guide

Remember that *the victory is in the Victory Guide*. Record your progress on My Progress Report located on page 22.

Week 8: *E* Is for Exercise

Bod4God Thought

It is better to exercise an hour a day than to be dead twenty-four hours a day.

Bod4God Memory Verse

Therefore, whether you eat or drink, or whatever you do, do all to the glory of God. (1 Corinthians 10:31)

Bod4God Reflection/Application Questions

1. First Corinthians 10:31 gives the basic principle by which believers are to determine their conduct. Everything we do must honor God. That is to be our motivation. In your opinion, how does a person exercise to the glory of God?

   ....

   ....

   ....

   ....

   ....

2. How would you describe your past exercise habits? Do they honor God? Explain.

   ....

   ....

   ....

....

....

3. In what ways are you physically active on a daily basis? What is your weekly exercise routine? Write your daily activity in the chart below.

Sun.	
Mon.	
Tues.	
Wed.	
Thurs.	
Fri.	
Sat.	

4. In 1 Timothy 4:8, Paul's emphasis is on godliness rather than physical exercise. Note that Paul is not downgrading the importance of physical exercise, just that he is emphasizing godliness. You cannot ignore one (godliness) to pursue the other (healthy body). Are you as concerned about godliness as you are about physical exercise?

....

....

....

....

....

5. In what ways are you exercising yourself to become more godly?

....

....

....

....

....

6. As I mentioned in this chapter, you have to set goals of input to achieve your goal of output. My output goal was to lose 100 pounds, while my input goals were all of the "small steps to life" I developed to meet the output goal of major weight loss. What is your output goal?

....

....

....

....

....

7. Have you written this goal down? If so, where will you post it so you can see it on a daily basis?

....

....

....

....

....

8. What input goals will you need to put in place to help you achieve your output goal?

....

....

....

....

....

9. Temptation will come. What are some of the greatest temptations you face in your struggle to become healthy? What are you doing to handle those difficult times?

....

....

....

....

....

10. After reading this chapter's Bod4God Close-Up, what can you relate to and what can you take from this person's story to apply to your own life and lifestyle plan?

....

....

....

....

....

Bod4God Small Steps
to Life Record

What "Skinny Things" Will You Do This Week?

Fill out this chart by indicating: (1) what you will do to eat less to live; (2) what you will do to exercise more to live; and (3) how many average daily ounces of water you will drink. Pick only a few things, and stick with them. Remember that weight loss and maintenance require you to *eat less* and *exercise more*.

Sun.	
Mon.	
Tues.	
Wed.	
Thurs.	
Fri.	
Sat.	

My Bod4God Journal

Teach me, O LORD, the way of Your statutes, and I shall keep it to the end.

Psalm 119:33

Record what God is telling you to do this week to apply the four keys to lasting weight loss.

Dedication: Honoring God with My Body

....

....

....

....

Inspiration: Motivating Myself for Change

....

....

....

....

....

Eat and Exercise: Managing My Habits

....

....

....

....

....

Team: Building My Circle of Support

....

....

....

....

....

T Is for Team:
A Personal Challenge

Don't Try to Lose Weight Alone;
Join a Team of Losers

Restore to me the joy of Your salvation, and uphold me by Your
generous Spirit.

Psalm 51:12

Let's talk some more about obesity. Physicians, weight trainers, and other
health personnel are talking more about Body Mass Index (BMI) than they
are the actual pounds that show up on the scale as gained or lost. That's
because muscle is heavier than fat, and the scale may be standing still if you
are increasing muscle by exercising. Even though you may weigh the same,
it could be that you are replacing fat with muscle. That's good, because
muscle burns fat. The higher the muscle to fat ratio in your body, the higher
your fat-burning metabolism. That's why men often have an advantage
over women in their ability to lose weight more quickly. Women can even
out that advantage by adding strength training to their aerobic exercise.

Everyone needs to know their BMI, and it is easy to calculate. There are
a number of BMI calculators on the internet. The one I like best is www
.cdc.gov/healthyweight/assessing/bmi/. There, you can enter your height and

weight and in an instant know what your BMI is. If your BMI is between 25 and 29, you are overweight. If it is more than 30, you are obese. Morbid obesity—sometimes called "clinically severe obesity"—is defined as being 100 pounds or more over ideal body weight or having a BMI of 40 or higher.

There is other valuable information on this website about the risks of being overweight or obese. There are ideas for helping you deal with your problem and even healthy recipes.

I want you to face the fact that you may be either overweight and headed toward obesity or obese and headed toward morbid obesity and certain death as a direct result. I am pleading with you to do something now—today—about your weight and unhealthy eating habits. Face reality and save your own life.

Perhaps you are not the one with the weight problem; perhaps you are the enabler who is helping your loved one stay obese. It's time for both of you to get honest and face the truth.

Obesity Is a Big Problem

Obesity has reached epidemic proportions in the United States. More than 2 in 3 adults are considered to be overweight or obese (with a BMI of greater than or equal to 25). Also, more than 1 in 3 can be diagnosed as obese (with a BMI greater than or equal to 30) and more than 1 in 20 adults have extreme obesity with a BMI of 40 or more. In addition, about one-third of children and adolescents ages six to nineteen are considered to be overweight or obese with more than 1 in 6 considered to be obese.[1] This trend toward obesity has been rapidly escalating for the last ten to fifteen years.

The worst offenders are in Middle America and the southeastern part of the country. According to the most recent data, 2 states have adult obesity rates above 35 percent, twenty states have rates at or above 30 percent, forty-three states have rates at or above 25 percent, and every state is above 20 percent. Mississippi and West Virginia have the highest rates of obesity at 35.1 percent, while Colorado has the lowest rate at 21.3 percent. All ten states with the highest rates of obesity are in the South or Midwest. Northeastern and western states comprise most of the states with the lowest rates of obesity. Between 2012 and 2013, six states showed statistically significant increases in adult obesity—Alaska, Delaware, Idaho, New Jersey, Tennessee, and Wyoming.[2] Are you shocked? You should be.

What's really sad is that this epidemic is preventable. Obesity is the most common preventable cause of death second only to smoking. It is the root cause of many medical conditions and is costing our society billions of dollars.

Overweight is defined as a body mass index (BMI) of 25 or higher, while obesity is defined as a BMI of 30 or higher. Research has shown that as people become overweight and obese their risk for developing the following conditions increases:

- Coronary heart disease
- Type 2 diabetes
- Cancers (endometrial, breast, and colon)
- Hypertension (high blood pressure)
- Dyslipidemia (for example, high total cholesterol or high levels of triglycerides)
- Stroke
- Liver and gallbladder disease
- Sleep apnea and breathing problems
- Osteoarthritis (a breakdown of cartilage and bone within a joint)
- Gynecological problems (abnormal periods, infertility)[3]

Why would any thinking person not do something about their obesity once these facts are presented? Is that super-sized meal, that four-layer chocolate cake, and those endless bowls of ice cream really worth your health? On the other hand, losing weight can cause you to live longer, have more energy, feel better, save money on both medical and pharmacy costs, and honor the Lord by taking care of the body He has given you.

Ask God to Be Your Personal Trainer

"But, Pastor Steve," I hear you whine, "I don't have anyone to work with. I don't have a team. I can't do this by myself." There are no excuses for not caring for your own body, the beautiful, finely tuned machine God gave you as your place of residence on earth. If you don't have anyone to work with, you are going to have to do it alone. Is it hard? Yes. Is it harder than working with a team to lose weight? Probably. But it can be done. I lost 70 pounds before we ever established the Losing To Live competitions. If I can do it, you can too.

That said, you have to have support for your weight-loss program even if you are doing it on your own. First, you have to get God on your team. I have a sneaking hunch that He has been hanging around waiting for you to get to this place. He wants your body to be all it can be. He has plans for you and for your life. He wants to help you.

Let's think of doing it alone as a team of one plus One—the second One being God Almighty who is able to do "above all that we ask or think" (Ephesians 3:20). Here are some Scriptures to help you through those tough times.

Put God on Your Team

Taste and see that the LORD is good; blessed is the man who trusts in Him! (Psalm 34:8)

Blessed are those who hunger and thirst for righteousness, for they shall be filled. (Matthew 5:6)

Live a Full Life in God

So I became great and excelled more than all who were before me in Jerusalem. Also, my wisdom remained with me. Whatever my eyes desired I did not keep from them. I did not withhold my heart from any pleasure. For my heart rejoiced in all my labor; and this was my reward from all my labor. Then I looked on all the works that my hands had done and on the labor in which I had toiled; and indeed all was vanity and grasping for the wind. There was no profit under the sun. (Ecclesiastes 2:9–11)

Rely on God for the Victory

If you faint in the day of adversity, your strength is small. (Proverbs 24:10)

I am the vine, you are the branches. He who abides in Me, and I in him, bears much fruit; for without Me you can do nothing. (John 15:5)

Pray Regularly

Call to Me, and I will answer you, and show you great and mighty things, which you do not know. (Jeremiah 33:3)

Men always ought to pray and not lose heart. (Luke 18:1)

Be Consistent in Daily Bible Reading

I have not departed from the commandment of His lips; I have treasured the words of His mouth more than my necessary food. (Job 23:12)

Your words were found, and I ate them, and Your word was to me the joy and rejoicing of my heart; for I am called by Your name, O LORD God of hosts. (Jeremiah 15:16)

Man shall not live by bread alone, but by every word that proceeds from the mouth of God. (Matthew 4:4)

Attend Church Weekly and Participate in Church Activities

I was glad when they said to me, "Let us go into the house of the LORD." (Psalm 122:1)

Let us consider one another in order to stir up love and good works, not forsaking the assembling of ourselves together, as is the manner of some, but exhorting one another, and so much the more as you see the Day approaching. (Hebrews 10:24–25)

The whole body, joined and knit together by what every joint supplies, according to the effective working by which every part does its share, causes growth of the body for the edifying of itself in love. (Ephesians 4:16)

Choose a Top-Notch Team

You must flex your teamwork muscles to be a big loser. The Bible says, "He who walks with wise men will be wise, but the companion of fools will be destroyed" (Proverbs 13:20). I had to choose wise people to be part of my team. I had to find people who would come alongside me as Aaron and Hur did for Moses, recorded in Exodus 17:12. Every time Moses held up his hands and stood for God, his team won the war. But when he dropped his hands because his arms were heavy, the team lost. Aaron and Hur came alongside to hold up his arms. Your team is crucial for winning the war on obesity. Who is going to hold up your hands?

I intentionally sought out people who could help me. There were three kinds of people I chose for my team.

People Who Will Educate You

I chose students of health. I read. I studied. I talked to people who had also lost weight. But first and foremost, I talked to my doctor. You must make a point to see a doctor before you begin any eating and exercise changes. My doctor played a major role in my weight loss and was always there to ask me how I was doing with my eating and exercising. For a long time I didn't have any good news to report to him. I was a diabetic, and I was supposed to see the doctor frequently. I didn't go because I didn't want him to tell me again and again what I should be doing and wasn't. Maybe you can relate to this. My doctor never backed down. He just kept asking. When I started exercising, he didn't tell me I was doing well to exercise three times a week. He said, "You eat every day, why don't you exercise every day?" I had to acknowledge he made a good point.

Read web pages, books, and articles written by people who can help you learn about good health. There is a huge amount of information available today, so there is no excuse for being ignorant about your health. "But books and magazines cost so much," I hear you protest. Think of this educational material as an investment in your own body. You are worth it! If money is tight, use the public library. You'll find plenty there to educate your mind about good health.

People Who Will Encourage You

Find some people who will encourage you. You need to have role models. I am so encouraged when I see all the people at Capital Baptist Church who have lost weight. I know this program—this lifestyle change—works, because I've seen it in action. If I were ever discouraged, all I'd have to do is sit down with Rich or Gail or any of the others and say, "Tell me your weight-loss story again," and I'd be encouraged to go on. It is truly amazing what these participants, with God's help, have done about getting their bodies back to health.

People Who Will Equip You

Finally, we all need people who will equip us—those who can show us how to do what we've purposed to do. Many people are the same as I was. They don't exercise. I think it would be great to have a personal trainer working with me on a regular basis, but I don't. However, the first time I went to the gym to exercise, a personal trainer took me around to show me the machines. He explained how to use each piece of equipment without injuring myself and told me what each piece of equipment would do to help me. He taught me how to build my endurance on each apparatus. That personal trainer had lost more than 100 pounds himself. I am thankful that he not only equipped me to work on the machines but also told me about nutritional items that have been a great help to me.

One other equipping help is the Body & Soul exercise program held at our church, which I mentioned earlier in the book. Perhaps joining such a program would work better for you than a gym workout. You have to find people and programs that can equip you for the long battle of losing weight. The good news is that after only a few days of exercise, you will begin to feel better than you have in a long time. That's something to look forward to right now.

A Team of Relationships

Of course, most important in my weight loss was that God and I were on the same side of the fence. In addition, I realized that I had to get my relationships across that fence too. I had to talk to my wife and kids and tell them what I was trying to do. I had to talk to my co-workers. I had to talk to my friends. I even had to talk to my mother. I couldn't have any of them sabotaging my plans for weight loss. You know, comments such as, "Just one piece of pie. You deserve it. You've worked so hard this week. And besides, I made it just for you."

I had to build a circle of support for my newfound journey to a healthy lifestyle. I had to ask for help. And that's not always easy for guys to do. I've learned that when a couple has a marriage problem, it's usually the wife who calls me for help. Guys, unfortunately, are embarrassed to ask for help. But, guys—I'm talking to you now—we have to get over it if we're going to get the support we need for our weight-loss program.

If you are planning to lose weight without the benefit of a team, first enlist God's help and then find yourself a partner. There is probably at least one other person in your circle of church friends who wants to lose weight too. Or maybe there's someone at your workplace. Set up a time when you email each other, get together, or talk on the phone about your victories or snags. Get a prayer partner to commit to praying for you on a daily basis. Share your successes with all your contacts and reward yourself—but not with food.

Let's go back to the Mayo Clinic website one more time to find their six strategies for success:

1. *Make a commitment.* Only you can make the commitment to treat your body better. External pressure from the people closest to you may scuttle your efforts to lose weight. You have to decide to lose weight to please yourself. It's a good idea to clear up any other major issues in your life so that you aren't distracted by them as you launch your weight-loss program.

2. *Get emotional support.* Pick people who want what's best for you and will encourage you. Find people who will listen to your concerns and feelings and who are willing to exercise with you for a healthier lifestyle.

3. *Set a realistic goal.* Aim to lose 1 to 2 pounds a week. You'll have to burn 500 to 1,000 more calories than you take in each day to accomplish this goal. Make your goals "process goals," such as exercising regularly, rather than "outcome goals," such as losing 50 pounds. Change your lifestyle by making "small steps to life."

4. *Learn to enjoy healthier foods.* Eat more plant-based foods such as fruits, vegetables, and whole grains. Strive for variety to help you achieve your goals without giving up taste or nutrition.

5. *Get active, stay active.* Cutting 500 calories from your daily diet can help you lose about a pound a week. But if you add a 45- to 60-minute brisk walk four days a week, you will double your rate of weight

loss. The goal of exercise is to burn calories. Even though regularly scheduled aerobic exercise is best for losing fat, any extra movement helps burn calories. Think about ways you can increase your physical activity throughout the day.

6. *Change your lifestyle* rather than considering yourself on a diet for a certain period of time. You have to make lifestyle changes that will remain in place all the way to the end of your life.[4]

Dealing with Those Who Doubt

Those who doubt are everywhere. And as soon as you get serious about losing weight, they come out of the woodwork and start saying things like, "So how many times have you been on a diet before?" and "Yoo-hoo, everybody, Pastor Steve's gonna get skinny. What do ya think about that? Think he can do it?" I'm not sure if it's jealousy that drives this kind of talk or an attitude or what. If you've been up and down in your weight as I have, maybe these folks really don't believe you can change. Come to think of it, why would they believe that this time will be different?

You just can't let them get to you. You have to realize it took you a while to get into this overweight situation and it's going to take a while to get out. People will begin to believe you are serious and will help you when they see you sticking to your small steps to life and that you are beginning to lose weight.

Spend some time reading the story of Daniel and think about the food choice he made. The king wanted Daniel to eat the richest foods the kingdom had to offer. He wanted Daniel to be healthy and thought that was the way to ensure his health. But Daniel knew something the king didn't. He knew the diet the king proposed would damage his health both physically and spiritually. Here's the story from *The Message:*

> But Daniel determined that he would not defile himself by eating the king's food or drinking his wine, so he asked the head of the palace staff to exempt him from the royal diet. The head of the palace staff, by God's grace, liked Daniel, but he warned him, "I'm afraid of what my master the king will do. He is the one who assigned this diet and if he sees that you are not as healthy as the rest, he'll have my head!"

But Daniel appealed to a steward who had been assigned by the head of the palace staff to be in charge of Daniel, Hananiah, Mishael, and Azariah: "Try us out for ten days on a simple diet of vegetables and water. Then compare us with the young men who eat from the royal menu. Make your decision on the basis of what you see."

The steward agreed to do it and fed them vegetables and water for ten days. At the end of the ten days they looked better and more robust than all the others who had been eating from the royal menu. So the steward continued to exempt them from the royal menu of food and drink and served them only vegetables. (Daniel 1:8–16)

The king represented someone negative in Daniel's life, and Daniel had to resolve to stick by his decision not to eat from the king's table. It worked. You, too, are going to have to deal with negative people, most of whom don't mean to be negative, but they truly can sabotage your plan. Also notice that in just ten days Daniel saw some results from healthy eating, and you can too!

What to Do about the Workplace

If ever there is a place to scuttle your weight-loss program, it is the workplace. Think about it. First, there are all the parties that happen during work hours. There are birthday parties, wedding and baby showers, retirement and welcoming parties, Christmas parties, and on and on it goes. Every one of them is a trap to set you back days in your efforts to eat healthy. Then there are the lunches and dinners out entertaining guests, and business trips on the company credit card that just beg you to spend money on a "really great" meal since the company is paying for it. The company may be paying money for the meal, but who is really paying for overeating and eating the wrong things? You are. If entertaining and eating out is a continuing lifestyle for you, you are probably wearing the result of workplace sabotage right around your middle.

What can you do about this serious problem in your health-conscious life? One thing you can do is watch what the skinny people at your company do. Do they load up on carbs at the event? Do they even eat? When eating out, do they eat the whole meal with appetizers included, or do they push back the plate when they've eaten half or less of the meal? Do they ask for a doggie bag? You can learn a lot from observing them.

Acknowledge that no one is forcing you to eat all the cookies, cakes, ice cream, and candy that show up at your workplace. You won't get your pay docked if you don't eat them. No one will twist your arm if you pass them by. Truly, most people won't pay any attention to whether you are eating the desserts or not. Be honest and admit that you are eating the junk food because you made a decision to eat it. You want it. Acknowledging that you have a problem is the first step to overcoming it.

Let's think of some ways to deal with this workplace problem.

- One thing you can do is make a game of the event to see how little you can eat and not have anyone notice.
- Take a small piece of cake or a cookie on a plate. Carry the plate around with you and keep talking to everyone. Don't eat what's on the plate; just carry it around. It will keep others from refilling your plate.
- Even better is to carry around a glass of punch, a soft drink, or a cup of coffee. You don't have to drink it. Just carry it around and when asked if you've had the dessert just say, "I'm fine with this," and indicate the drink.
- Think about what the purpose of the event is. Usually it is to honor someone. So instead of eating, spend the time talking to the honoree and other guests. It will make you very popular as a guest.
- Leave as quickly as you can and reduce the temptation to eat by simply walking away from it.
- Don't volunteer to help clean up unless you have been assigned that task. There is too much temptation to nibble the leftovers.
- If you are planning the party, be sure to include some snack trays with veggies and fruit with low-fat and/or sugar-free dips and dressings for yourself and the others who are eating healthy as well.
- Eat a small healthy snack before you go to the event. A handful of almonds is a good choice.
- Get active. Part of the problem of weight gain at the office is the inactivity of sitting behind a desk all day. There are some great exercises

you can do right at your desk. Set a timer to remind you to do these simple exercises:

1. For your tummy: Sit tall and straighten the spine. Then clench the abdominal muscles as tightly as possible, pulling your belly button back toward the spine. Hold for one to five seconds and repeat twenty times. Do at least three times daily.

2. For your thighs: While seated with your knees together, imagine someone is pulling them apart and it's your job to keep them together by squeezing your inner thigh muscles in one-second pulses. Do this at least three times daily.

3. For your backside: Start to stand up, with heels digging into the ground to contract the backside muscles, but pause a beat about three-quarters of the way through the standing motion. Sit back down, and then, finally stand up as you normally would. It's a great way to get exercise without even breaking a sweat.

- Better yet, go for a walk on your lunch break. Keep a pair of walking shoes under your desk.

I hope you see now that even if you don't have a group competition or an established group to help you, you can still be a team of one and ask God to join you in this very important battle for your body and your future. He is just waiting for you to ask for His help, and He will bring resources to you of which you have never dreamed.

A Bod4God Close-Up

The "Big Guy" No More

Brian Sumner
Lost 115 pounds

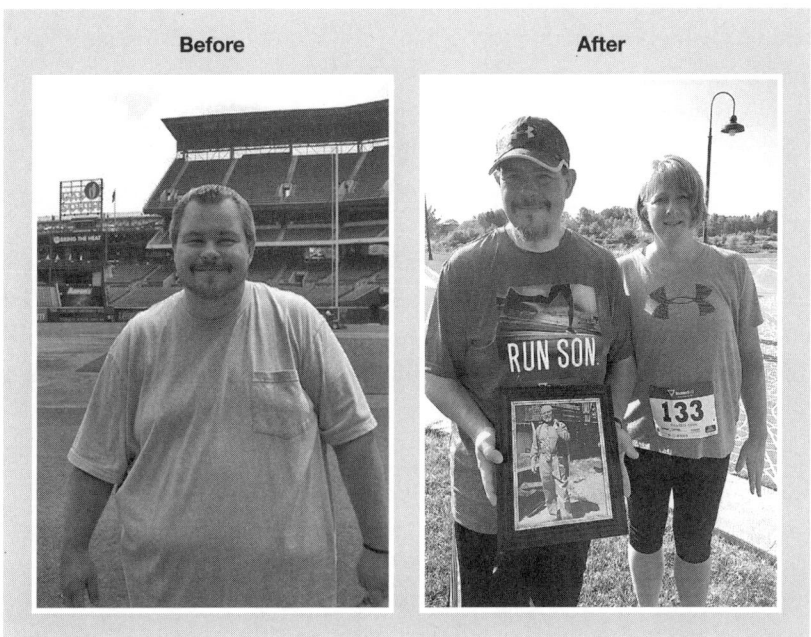

Before
After

For most of my life, I was labeled the "big guy." Over the past thirty years, I probably lost 125 pounds, all of which I put back on and then some. I watched my dad, who wasn't as big as I was, struggle with diabetes and heart issues, and I knew I was headed down the same road. I started experiencing health problems like high blood pressure and cholesterol, and my knees were suffering from the pressure of all my excess weight. I thought I would have to learn to live with all of these conditions, and I saw no hope for me to ever lose weight. However, something clicked about two years ago when I realized I was going to die if I didn't take action and make some drastic changes in my life and health. At 355 pounds, my weight was becoming something I could no longer ignore.

My inspiration for change came from my dad. I love and miss him so much. Unfortunately, I lost him to a stroke. He was only sixty-seven years old. I didn't expect to lose him so early. I knew that I wanted to be around for my family for a long time, and I desperately wanted to be healthy. From the beginning, my goal was not about an amount of pounds lost. That to me is short-term thinking. My goal was to live a healthy lifestyle for the rest of my life. I wanted to live. Thankfully, I have had great mentors and encouragers on this journey, like Pastor Steve Reynolds. I am a radio host, and I've interviewed him for years on the radio about *Bod4God*, but I always felt a little hypocritical because my health was in such terrible shape. But now, his book has been a tremendous influence on me, and has helped me achieve my health goals.

Through a lot of hard work, I have been able to lose 115 pounds. At forty-eight years old, I have more energy than I've had in years, and more energy makes it easier for me to be a better servant. I now view my exercise and working out as an act of worship to God, and I am more concerned about being a good steward of the body He gave me.

One of the things that has helped me lose the weight is maintaining portion control. I pay much more attention to the amount of food I am eating, and I do not go back for seconds. I also eat slower and drink lots of water. It is amazing to me that I now actually crave water. I used to hate exercising because I always thought short term. My old philosophy was to jog or run to lose weight, and then once I lost the weight I would quit. Now, I love to exercise. It has become a source of stress relief, and I feel much better after. I have found things I enjoy doing, and I work out with my wife. Having someone on the journey with me is a huge help. I love what Pastor Steve says about exercise being a habit, a sacred appointment you keep with yourself. I have really taken that to heart.

One of my biggest struggles is not getting discouraged when I step on the scale and don't see the pounds coming off. I try not to be a slave to the scale because in the past, this has stopped me from being consistent in my exercise and healthy eating choices. I would think to myself, *I'm not losing, so I might as well quit.* I have learned to keep my mind focused on the long term, to keep making the best food choices I can, and to remember that it took thirty years to get in bad shape. I focus on the fact that change is happening, but it isn't going to happen overnight.

Pastor Steve's book *Bod4God* is a must-have for me. I have marked it from cover to cover and refer to it often. I also mentor others on their health journey and recommend the book and pull advice from it all the time. I am so thankful for Pastor Steve's wisdom and that he shared his story with me and the world.

I tell people all the time to just start making healthy changes and not to compare their journey to someone else's. This is your race. Put all your energy into getting healthy, reaching out to others, praying often, and finding something you enjoy doing. We all stumble and fall. That's life. But don't stay down—get up again and continue.

This is a lifelong journey for me and since starting, this is the best I have felt in years. I have more energy, am less stressed, and I feel closer to God through the act of worshiping Him with my whole life and body. My new motto is "Sweat is fat crying," and I love to see it weep! I keep reminding myself of lifetime change, lifestyle change. I didn't get to over 300 pounds overnight, and it's going to take time to lose it. There are no magic pills or shortcuts. My answer to people when they ask me how I have done it is to eat less and exercise more. Thanks for allowing me a chance to share my story with you. Now it's your turn to start working on your story.

Small Steps to Life Ideas

Remember, Rome wasn't built in a day, and neither will your new body be built in a day or even a week or month. But little by little you will lay a new foundation for your new body, and little by little you will build new eating and exercise habits on that foundation; and one day, you'll look in the mirror at a new you. You can do this!

What Do You Need to Know about H_2O?

I start drinking a lot of water first thing in the morning and drink water all day long as my main beverage. I may vary what I drink in the evening. I also eat lots of fruits and vegetables that have a high water content.

Small Food Step

Eat breakfast. Eating breakfast gets your metabolism going for the day. That gives you more energy. If you skip breakfast, you set yourself up to snack during the morning, often on high-fat foods (donuts and sweet rolls). Missing breakfast can also cause you to eat too much food later in the day at other meals.

- Eating breakfast every day may reduce the risk for obesity and insulin resistance syndrome—an early sign of developing diabetes—by as much as 35 to 50 percent, according to a study presented at a recent American Heart Association conference.
- Eat whole-grain cereal. Look for cereals that list whole grain or bran as their first ingredient and contain at least 2 grams of dietary fiber per serving. Bran cereal and oatmeal contain at least 7 grams per serving, or about 25 percent of the recommended daily intake. Fiber One cereal contains 15 grams of fiber for a half cup.
- No time is not an excuse. Here's a quick way to make oatmeal—a great breakfast cereal. Pour one cup of water in a good-sized micro-wavable bowl (the cereal bubbles up when cooking). Add a half cup of

old-fashioned oats (steel cut are the best). Just don't use instant, as they turn into something resembling wallpaper paste. Add a tablespoon of raisins or other dried fruit. You can add cinnamon, nutmeg, or maple flavoring (not maple syrup). Microwave for two to three minutes; however, cooking times may vary, so adjust as needed. You can add a few almonds, skim milk, or low-fat soy milk. It doesn't get much faster than that for a quick, hot, nourishing breakfast.

- If cereal is not for you first thing in the morning, make a fruit smoothie with yogurt. Or have low-fat cheese and whole-grain crackers. Peanut butter spread on whole-wheat toast or a bagel fills you up.
- Search the fridge for leftovers that are tasty and nutritious. Who says you can't eat stir-fry in the morning, or a slice of whole-wheat vegetarian pizza?

Small Exercise Step

If you work at a desk, try the exercises given on page 202. Some call these "deskercises." These days, many exercise programs offer chair options. Other ideas include:

- Buy an aerobic or other kind of exercise DVD and begin working out with it. You don't have to spend a lot of money. You can find many such DVDs in thrift shops and places that resell them.
- Your local library offers all sorts of free health information, including exercise books.

Bod4God Victory Guide

Remember that *the victory is in the Victory Guide*. Record your progress on My Progress Report located on page 22.

Week 9: *T* Is for Team: A Personal Challenge

Bod4God Thought

Don't try to lose weight alone; join a team of losers.

Bod4God Memory Verse

Restore to me the joy of Your salvation, and uphold me by Your generous Spirit. (Psalm 51:12)

Bod4God Reflection/Application Questions

1. In what way does Psalm 51:12 give you motivation in continuing with your Bod4God lifestyle plan?

   ....

   ....

   ....

   ....

   ....

2. Proverbs 13:20 says that if we want to be wise, we need to walk with wise people. Who should be part of your team? (Remember, there are people on my team I have never met personally, but they have educated, encouraged, and equipped me.) Write the names of these people below.

   People who will educate you:

   ....

   ....

....

....

People who will encourage you:

....

....

....

....

People who will equip you:

....

....

....

....

3. Can you identify someone who might be negative about your attempt to lose weight? What will you do to deal with that negativity?

....

....

....

....

4. Read Matthew 18:15. What techniques does this Scripture offer as a way to handle negative people?

....

....

....

....

....

5. Read Daniel 1. What techniques does this Scripture offer as a way to handle negative people?

....

....

....

....

....

6. What do you need to do to avoid temptation in your workplace?

....

....

....

....

....

7. After reading this chapter's Bod4God Close-Up, what can you relate to and what can you take from this person's story to apply to your own life and lifestyle plan?

....

....

....

....

....

Bod4God Small Steps
to Life Record

What "Skinny Things" Will You Do This Week?

Fill out this chart by indicating: (1) what you will do to eat less to live, (2) what you will do to exercise more to live; and (3) how many average daily ounces of water you will drink. Pick only a few things, and stick with them. Remember that weight loss and maintenance require you to *eat less* and *exercise more*.

Sun.	
Mon.	
Tues.	
Wed.	
Thurs.	
Fri.	
Sat.	

My Bod4God Journal

Teach me, O LORD, the way of Your statutes, and I shall keep it to the end.

Psalm 119:33

Record what God is telling you to do this week to apply the four keys to lasting weight loss.

Dedication: Honoring God with My Body

....

....

....

....

Inspiration: Motivating Myself for Change

....

....

....

....

Eat and Exercise: Managing My Habits

....

....

....

....

Team: Building My Circle of Support

....

....

....

....

....

T Is for Team:
A Group Competition

Christians Don't Smoke Pot,
but They Do a Lot of Potlucks

Two are better than one, because they have a good reward for
their labor.

Ecclesiastes 4:9

Why can't the local church be a place where people learn how to live healthy
lives and lose weight? The Bible clearly commands Christians to have a
Bod4God, and local churches must help people in this area. My desire is
to help Christians become the most fit group of people in America, not
the fattest. I have a vision of entire churches full of Bod4God losers all
over our country. When I preached the "Bod4God: Four Keys to a Better
Body" sermon series at Capital Baptist Church, my goal was to motivate
our congregation to become the biggest group of losers in the United
States. We have lost over 24,000 pounds—that is over 12 tons of weight
loss so far—and we are still losing. I would like to tell you about our first
competition and what we are currently doing as well as how you can set
up a competition in your church (see also appendix D).

I knew that a sermon series alone wasn't going to help people get to their weight goals. So, coinciding with the series, we launched the Losing To Live Weight Loss Competition as an opportunity for people to lose weight in a fun, supportive environment. It was a natural outflow of the "Team" key. I wanted to give others the same kind of team support and motivation I had received from my own group of encouragers.

What I found after experiencing this competition was that the 150 people who joined the competition—a large percentage of whom weren't members of our church—became my encouragement, motivation, and inspiration. I felt as if they had come alongside me in making a difference for me, for themselves, and for so many people all around them.

To open up the plan to those outside our congregation (as an outreach and a ministry to them), we advertised on local radio and with brochures and an announcement on the church's marquee. Our materials offered this invitation: "Don't try to lose weight by yourself. Join a team of losers at Capital Baptist Church."

With the media attention from the *Washington Post* and local and national (later, even international) TV, people came in droves to find out what would motivate a Baptist pastor to take such a personal interest in his congregation's physical health. Then, when FOX News's Neil Cavuto labeled me the "anti-fat pastor," it certainly got people's attention. I believe God allowed this to happen to launch what has now become a national movement of losers through Bod4God.

We kicked off our first competition on Sunday, January 14, 2007, with—of all things—an orientation luncheon. I shared the details of the competition and invited people to participate. A professional chef, and member of our church, prepared a beautiful (and delicious) healthy spread: lots of vegetables and tasty salads along with a "wrap bar" that let participants choose healthy meats, cheeses, and veggies to fold into their own soft tortilla wrappers.

The opening was a great rah-rah event, and dozens of people found themselves surprised that they were enjoying the healthy fare every bit as much as their old unhealthy choices. This was the first among countless successes experienced by participants, who lost a total of 1,310 pounds.

One of our Losing To Live participants lost 24 pounds. She says, "I was on a low-fat diet for ten years and didn't lose weight. I joined a gym and went for two years. Still no loss. It just wasn't happening." But she is now successful, and she credits her success this time to being part of a Losing To Live team. "I needed a group to hold me accountable. It was a combination of things. First, I had to dedicate my weight to God, and then, I had to lose weight to God's glory. The team provided the extra oomph I needed—the accountability of our whole group—to lose weight."

What Happens at a Weekly Meeting

Each week during a competition, competitors have the opportunity to weigh in (in private, using a good scale) on Saturday, during each of our three Sunday morning services, as well as before and after our Sunday evening competition group meetings.

At the big gathering in the church auditorium on Sunday evening, we open the session by announcing our weight-loss results and celebrating each team's achievements of the previous week. This is an inspiring time as the teams—each having chosen a fruit name (lemon and passion fruit) or a vegetable name (squash and rutabaga)—celebrate their total team weight-loss percentages. Individuals on the teams also compete to become one of the top ten losers.

Input from Experts

After the cheerleading session, we provide information to the entire group through showing a Bod4God video or through a live speaker. The Bod4God videos are available in the Bod4God DVD series, which also includes group starter tools (available at www.bod4god.org). They are designed to be a perfect complement to this book. There are twelve twenty-five-minute video sessions to go with each chapter of the book. Each one includes a talk from me and expert interviews with doctors, trainers, nutritionists, and pastors as well as testimonies from Bod4God big losers and participants. They also include twelve Bod4God thoughts and twenty-four Bod4God factoids. The goal is to provide information to motivate and equip competitors to move forward with their healthy lifestyle choices.

Sometimes we invite health experts to speak to the entire group. One week, for example, a board certified internal medicine physician in our congregation, Liz Berbano, might give us an update on the latest medical research on how to fight back against obesity. Another week a certified internist might come to speak and to offer baseline blood work (glucose and cholesterol) and blood pressure readings for a nominal fee for any competitor who wishes to participate.

Another week someone like Vivian Hutson, a registered dietician from our congregation, might be a guest speaker. Vivian has become key to our program, as she directs the weighing in of each participant week after week, offering encouragement and challenging them when needed. Vivian has a great story. She's been involved as a key player in creating our church's health ministry plan. Her training gives her a unique perspective to offer competitors and the knowledge on how best to motivate them.

Vivian found the weigh-in times were great opportunities to get to know people and listen to their deeper needs. "They don't just want to talk about their diets. They also tell me if they've had a stressful week; they promise to do better," she says. But Vivian is careful never to be judgmental—even when someone has a gainer week. "I ask them what they wish they had done differently. Then I challenge them to put it behind them. That was last week! Now let's make healthy lifestyle choices for this week." And, of course, Vivian helps them focus on God rather than the stress or unhappiness of the previous week. "We pray to have a healthier body, not just for self-gratification but for God."

Vivian and her team keep the records to update our database each week—her logs help track individual and team weight loss by pounds and by percentage using a Microsoft Excel spreadsheet. She comments, "When I teach other community nutrition classes, I never see the success I see in this program. I think what we see here will last for a long time because they are doing it for God—for the right reason."

Team Time

But the big group sessions are just the beginning. Most competitors connect with the program when they break into their small group teams. They begin by naming themselves a fruit or vegetable. In their small group they go over the information in this book and specifically discuss the weekly Victory Guide assignments.

This is a nonthreatening time to interact with the material, to share ideas on what works and what doesn't work for each person. We cheer for successes. We encourage where needed, and, most of all, we pray with each other. The teams build relationships so strong that members pray for one another all week long. Some call or email each other to keep lines of communication open between the Sunday meetings. For most participants, the team time is the highlight of the program because they attribute their weight-loss success and much of their spiritual growth to their team relationships.

Exercise Time

In regard to exercise, we have a variety of walking groups and beginner exercise programs. We also partner closely with a wonderful ministry called Body & Soul (www.bodyandsoul.org). The Body & Soul team offers group exercise four times a week with weekday, evening, and weekend options. I love this program because each session contains elements of spiritual and physical exercise. The cardio and strength training to contemporary Christian music provides an inspirational, safe, modest setting where people of all ages and abilities can work out together in a nonthreatening environment—while filling their minds with biblical messages.

Victory Celebration

The competition concludes with a victory celebration. It is a very exciting event. The joyous emotion in the room is incredible. The individual teams first gather together to discuss the content of week 12 in this book. After this special time, all the teams gather together to celebrate their overall weight-loss results and to announce our biggest losing team and individual loser.

A Big Finish!

With such a winning program going on for so many weeks, we wanted to plan a big finale for our first competition—one that would top our opening luncheon and yet be consistent with all the Bod4God progress we'd all made. We planned a 5K run/walk. We advertised and opened it up to the community. It was a program wrap-up, a celebration, and a community outreach—all rolled into one.

The 5K path started and ended on our church property, and we were able to get professional runners to help establish the route. We walked the route several Sunday evenings before the event, and we enlisted volunteers from the congregation to help along the route on race day. We found a number of corporate sponsors to donate prizes and products for the event, and after a few planning meetings, we were ready to run the race.

Finally, when race day came, 350 people participated, many of whom were among the 150 Losing To Live competitors and many more who were from the community at large. It was an event deemed a success by all.

Competitor Damon Johnson said, "My wife, Charlene, and I enjoyed the fellowship, running for Jesus against obesity, and the healthy brunch you provided for all of us. Keep on encouraging all God's people to be the best that God wants them to be and inspiring them all to enjoy eating healthy, exercising, and staying faithful to the Lord by doing His will."

The Losing To Live 5K Run/Walk is now an annual event at our church.

A Model for a Team Competition

I want to share with you some details for how you can start a team competition in your church or organization.

How to Get Started

Starting a Losing To Live Competition ministry can be a very rewarding experience! Everywhere you look these days—on television, in books, and newspaper articles—a main topic of conversation seems to be in health and weight loss. If you have a burden to address the issue of good health and weight loss with those you come in contact with, especially in your local church or another organization, then why not start a Losing To Live team competition ministry?

So you might ask, "How do I get started?" First, commit the matter to prayer. Be sure to follow God's lead and not your own. Also ask around to see if there are people interested in such a program.

The next step is to meet with your pastor or appointed leader. Communicate the need for the program in your local church. When your pastor is out in the community, they probably notice that there are a lot of people who are overweight. There certainly are people in your own congregation who suffer from obesity. This really is a *growing* problem and needs to be addressed not just by the media outlets but by the churches. Make sure your pastor is aware that Christians are the most overweight people group in America.

Share with the pastor the fact that Losing To Live was developed through much Bible study and prayer by Pastor Steve Reynolds, who weighed over 340 pounds and was diagnosed with high blood pressure, high cholesterol, and diabetes. Through following biblical principles, Pastor Reynolds lost more than 100 pounds and no longer has these diseases. Explain that Losing To Live will show people how to lose weight and keep it off through establishing a Bod4God lifestyle. Highlight the four keys to this program, which are:

1. Dedication: Honoring God with Your Body
2. Inspiration: Motivating Yourself for Change
3. Eat and Exercise: Managing Your Habits
4. Team: Building Your Circle of Support

Next, communicate the benefits of the program. The program is biblically based, which means that participants will be spending more time in God's Word. It's an opportunity for church members to work as a team to achieve good health. Also, people who may otherwise speak only in passing will have a chance to build relationships through time spent together in a group setting.

Another great benefit of the program is its appeal to people outside the church. What an opportunity for outreach. So many people have tried all the other diet plans and failed. For those people, a God-centered plan would be a new approach to an age-old problem. Also, there are people with questions about God who have no desire to attend church but would become involved in a weight-loss program. The exposure to godly principles could spark a desire to learn more about God. This could eventually lead to an increase in church participation from the surrounding community.

You must consider the space you'll need and its availability. You will need adequate space at the church, or wherever you meet. You'll need to discuss what days and the times you can meet. Share that participants will meet once a week for twelve weeks and that each session will last for 90 minutes. You will need a space for all the participants to meet together for the first 30 minutes, a place for the individual teams to meet together for the final hour, and a private place to put your scale for the weigh-in.

Explain that the funds for the materials will be recovered from the participants. Each participant should obtain the official Losing To Live Participant Kit, which includes the *Bod4God* book, Losing To Live T-shirt, and refrigerator magnet. This kit can be purchased at www.bod4god.org and can be ordered in bulk by the leader of the competition, or each participant can order their own kit directly from the Bod4God website.

Then ask your pastor to endorse the program from the pulpit and possibly through personal participation. Most people will follow their leader. If the pastor doesn't want to be involved, ask if they will allow you to develop a Losing To Live team challenge in the church and recruit others who may be interested.

Allow your pastor time to consider this ministry and pray about it, and then follow up. If the pastor says no, then respect that decision. If the pastor says yes, then make it happen. Follow the step-by-step guide for a successful group competition in appendix D (pages 275–79).

What It Takes to Lead a Group of "Losers"

In Luke 6:39–40, Jesus says, "Can the blind lead the blind? Will they not both fall into the ditch? A disciple is not above his teacher, but everyone who is perfectly trained will be like his teacher." Here are some tips to help you be a good leader.

Key Information for Key Leaders

Here is some key information for those who will be leading a team of "losers":

- The number one law of leadership is that everything rises and falls on the quality of the leadership. If you have volunteered to lead a team, spend some time in prayer about the responsibility you have taken on. How can you make your leadership sparkle and light the way for the participants on your team?
- Success in our program is measured primarily by weight loss.
- Losing To Live exists to teach people how to lose weight and keep it off through a Bod4God lifestyle. This includes four keys to lasting weight

loss: (1) Dedication: Honoring God with your body; (2) Inspiration: Motivating yourself for change; (3) Eat and Exercise: Managing your habits; (4) Team: Building your circle of support.

Team Captain Responsibilities

Here are four ways to help your team lose if you are chosen as a team captain:

1. Lead your team by example, modeling the four keys to lasting weight loss.
2. Oversee your team by following the best practices.
3. Study and prayerfully prepare for your team meetings.
4. Encourage your team through regular communications.

Meeting Schedule

Weekly team meetings at our church are held on Sunday night from 6:00 to 7:30 p.m.; however, group meetings can happen anywhere, at any time, and on any day. The format for our meetings is as follows:

- 6:00 to 6:30 p.m. We meet as one group for information and sit together as teams. We announce our overall total competition and weekly weight loss, and our top competition and weekly losing team and individual loser. We show a Bod4God DVD or have an expert speak on a health topic, especially as it relates to weight loss.
- 6:30 to 7:30 p. m. We meet for inspiration as individual teams in classrooms. The focus during this time is going over the material in this book and other books, particularly the weekly Victory Guide assignment.

Weigh-In Procedure

Weigh-ins are done on Saturday mornings, Sunday mornings, and on Sunday nights before and after the Losing To Live meeting. Every competitor is asked to weigh in at least eight times during the competition. We ensure that each competitor has privacy during their weigh-in.

Each week the team captains are emailed a report showing the individual and team results from the weigh-in. In addition, each week during our opening time in the auditorium we report on the top three team losers and top ten individual losers. This helps maintain overall motivation and encouragement, both as a team and as individuals.

The weight-loss competition is based on the *percentage* of weight loss, not the *amount* of weight loss.

Weekly Assignments

Participants read this book and other books each week. We give out weekly assignments in order to keep participants on track in completing the book study.

Group Rules

There are two basic group rules. First, the confidentiality rule: What is shared in the group stays in the group (unless permission is given to share the information outside of the group). Second, the conversation rule: You can only participate in the group discussion if you did the weekly assignment. Otherwise, you must just listen to others.

What to Do Next

Once you complete Bod4God, your goal should be to establish an ongoing wellness ministry. Today, our Losing To Live Weight Loss Competition offers four levels.

Level one, first-time participants go through my first book, *Bod4God: Twelve Weeks to Lasting Weight Loss*. Many people like to go through this book twice before moving on to the next level.

Level two participants go through my book *Get Off The Couch: 6 Motivators to Help You Lose Weight and Start Living*. This book is the perfect follow-up to *Bod4God. Get Off the Couch* will help you:

- Win the battle against overeating and take control of food cravings with God's strength.
- Increase your energy to perform better at work, play with your kids, and enjoy time with your spouse.

- Boost your confidence and feel better when you look in the mirror.
- Lose weight and keep it off!

This book is another critical and helpful step to lasting weight loss.

Level three participants go through a First Place 4 Health Bible Study. Level four is our weight maintenance level for those who have reached their ideal weight, and they also go through a First Place 4 Health Bible Study.

First Place 4 Health is a faith-based weight-loss plan supported and endorsed by registered dietitians and physicians with a mission to provide a biblical wellness program that enables individuals to achieve balance in spirit, soul, mind, and body based on giving Christ first place. Based on proven techniques and more than thirty years of experience, First Place 4 Health is the most complete Christ-centered healthy living program available. The program will help you create balance in the four core areas of your life—emotional, spiritual, mental, and physical. The results? Weight loss and total health from the inside out!

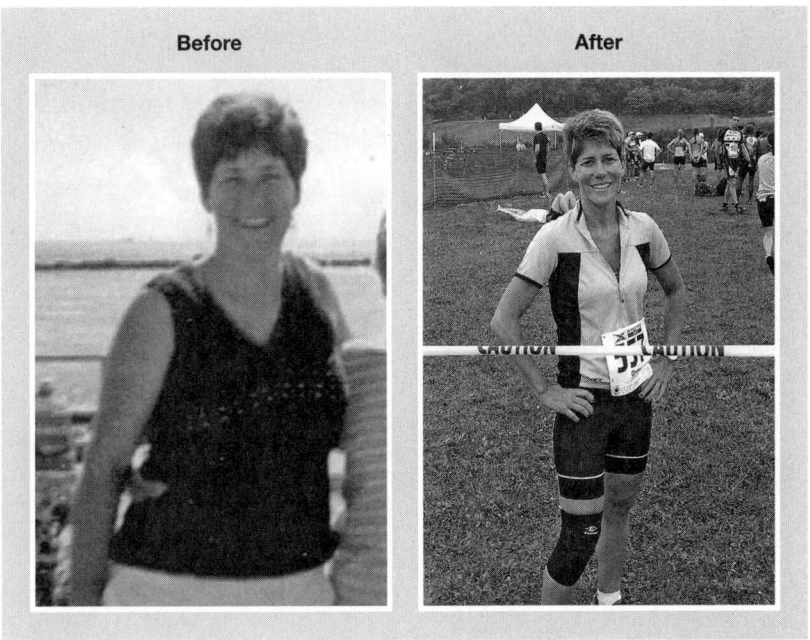

Before   **After**

The following success story from Becky Stephenson, a woman who participated in the First Place 4 Health program, portrays the healthy lifestyles that result from the practical disciplines of the program:

When people see me, they automatically think I have been in shape and exercised all my life, but that is so far from the truth, which is that I loved to eat and was a couch potato. I knew every number on the fast-food menus and had such a sweet tooth that dessert was part of each meal. I was so out of shape and overweight that my arms used to flap every time I moved them.

My eating and non-exercise habits led me to years of yo-yo dieting. I tried so many diets, none of which worked. I would lose 20 pounds but would then go back to my old eating habits and gain it all back again. I lost the same 20 pounds at least four times in my life.

By the time I was forty-four, I was overweight by 30-plus pounds, spiritually dry, and depressed. I knew I needed to change my life, but I didn't know in what direction to go. I was on high blood pressure meds and wasn't able to walk up a flight of steps without being short of breath. My church was offering a First Place 4 Health class, and I felt the Lord leading me to sign up.

The class changed my life. Through the Bible study, I realized how much God loved me and that He had plans for my life. I knew He wanted me to be free of the obsession I had for food and my avoidance for exercise.

God says He will restore what the locusts have eaten (Joel 2:25), and that is what He has done in my life. I feel better now than I did in my twenties and am doing things I never dreamed of doing. I can now run up a flight of steps without getting short of breath, and every time I hit the top I always praise God. I also went from a size 10 to a size 2.

I am now preparing for an Ironman Triathlon. I went from being a couch potato to placing second in a Duathlon, which is a 56-mile bike ride climbing over 6 thousand feet, then a 13.1 mile run on one of the toughest courses in the world. God is so amazing.

I just want to encourage you that it's never too late and you're never too old or out of shape to get started. When I started biking, I had to walk up every hill in my neighborhood, and when I started to run, it was a few feet at a time. I was never an athlete, so I started from the beginning—one step at a time. I remember reading in one of Carole Lewis's books about an old Chinese proverb, "The journey of a thousand miles begins with a single step."

My step started with the First Place 4 Health Bible study, and then God did the rest. As I put Him first, He balanced the rest of my life. His Word tells us that apart from Him we can do nothing (John 15:5). It's amazing to see where God has brought me, and I give all the glory to Him. I pray that God will take first place in your life as well. [1]

Start a Losing To Live Weight Loss Competition

Ecclesiastes 4:9–12 tells us that teamwork produces (1) mutual success, (2) mutual support, and (3) mutual strength. Your participation in the Losing To Live Weight Loss Competition will allow you to experience the power of teamwork as related to your health and weight loss.

Teamwork through a Losing To Live competition produces tremendous results. We do three competitions a year in our church, and we have now lost more than 24,000 pounds—that is over 12 tons of weight loss. Many other churches and organizations are doing this competition and are seeing tremendous results.

I urge you to start this program in your church or organization and help me change lives one pound at a time.

For more information or to get the Bod4God DVD series, which also includes group starter tools (such as forms and promotional helps), please visit www.bod4god.org or contact me at the following:

Losing To Live
P.O. Box 300
Merrifield, VA 22116
703-635-7100 • 866-596-6008

God never meant for us to go through life alone. He created us for community so we can encourage and edify one another and keep each other on track. The same principle applies to weight loss. I believe that it is much easier to achieve lasting weight loss when you are committed to a team of people with the same goal. So join a team of losers today, commit yourself to the twelve-week program that will help you lose weight and keep it off, and see what God can do in your life and in your health. Start losing so that you can start living!

A Bod4God Close-Up

Move It and Lose It

Tamara Cothrell
Lost 75 pounds

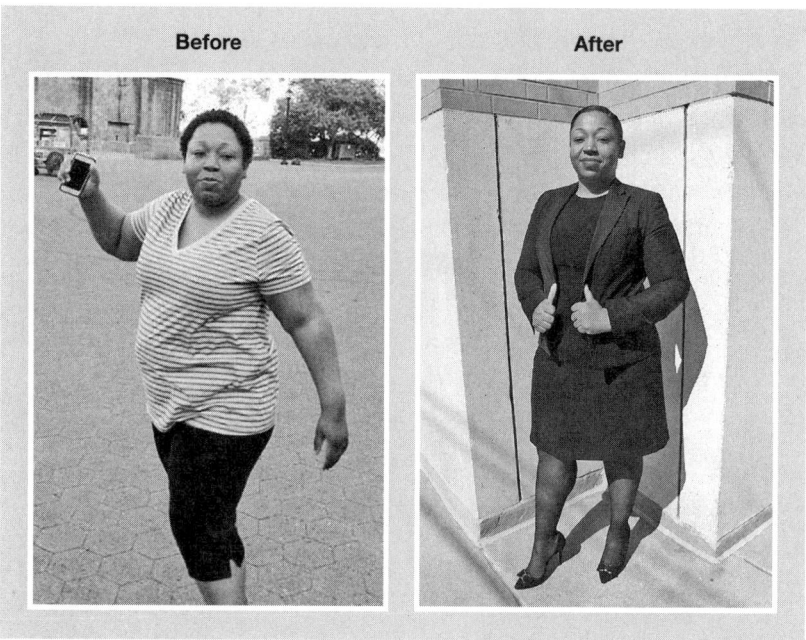

Before | After

Since having children, I have struggled with weight. During a physical examination my doctor told me that I was entering the pre-diabetic range. At the age of thirty-four, I weighed 271 pounds. Feeling shattered and defeated, I knew something had to change because my children needed their mom around. So I started walking .25 mile in my community. I was winded and could barely stand up at the end of this brief walk. How embarrassing! But I didn't care what anybody thought of me and my weight. Each time I walked I would try to increase my distance. At the end of the month, I was up to .5 mile. I started to feel the difference in being able to walk longer.

While attending Capital Baptist Church in Annandale, Virginia, one Sunday, I saw the advertisement for the Losing To Live competition and thought to myself, *How groundbreaking would it be if I actually lost weight using the principles of the Bible?* Little did I know that my life was about to change.

I showed up on the first night and weighed in. I got my *Bod4God* book and Losing To Live T-shirt and joined my team. We called ourselves "The Fighting Figs" (Losing To Live teams name themselves after a fruit or vegetable). Having the team made all the difference. We motivated each other and shared tips on making small steps to life. These small changes were not drastic, and I didn't think making them would have an impact on my weight loss. Well, I was wrong! I went on to lose over 20 pounds, and I finished in the top ten in the overall competition. I knew I was going to keep going. My Losing To Live T-shirt became my inspiration. When I put it on, I felt accountable to my team. They motivated me so much that every time I worked out I made sure I had on my T-shirt. I even took the shirt with me on my mission trip to Saltillo, Mexico, as a reminder that no matter where in the world I am, I need to make better choices. I also made sure I was getting sufficient activity while I was in Mexico.

I loved my team. I also followed the Losing To Live Facebook page, and on the days when I felt like giving up, a message would pop up in my timeline about making small changes or a Scripture verse was there to inspire me. So I kept pushing to lose more weight. I decided to get a trainer after I was unable to get out of the plateau I was experiencing. I lost even more weight, and now I focus on building muscle, burning fat, and lowering my BMI. I work out six to seven days a week, meeting with my trainer twice per week for strength training. I am so proud to share with you that I have lost 75 pounds since I started this health journey.

My small steps to life were simple changes, ones that anyone can do. I stopped using salt, drank half my body weight in ounces of water almost every day, and started to control my portions. One key thing that I learned over the course of my health journey thus far is that I have to eat real food to lose weight, no starvation, no gimmicks, just eat like my grandmother did. The *Bod4God* book was a godsend because I had tried everything else to lose weight, but I never thought about using the Bible as my guide and really applying the principles to my life. Pastor Reynolds shared his small changes and foods he had started eating, and I started buying those foods as well. I follow his tips and menu items because it has made my life easier and took the guesswork out of trying to figure out what to eat. I also invested in a pedometer and did some form of physical activity every day.

I work in Washington, DC, so I use the subway to commute. Instead of using the metro stop closest to my office, I instead got off four metro stops away. This helped me walk 3.5 miles per day in addition to taking the steps and finding creative ways to move while I worked. My team also helped me by sharing what small steps to life they were making in exercise. My initial goal on my pedometer was 7,000 steps per day. Then one team member came in and said they were making 10,000 steps per day their goal. Being the competitor that I am, I increased my daily goal to 10,000 steps as well.

Keeping a healthy mind-set is still a struggle. However, I focus on Romans 12:2, which says, "And do not be conformed to this world, but be transformed by the renewing of your mind, that you may prove what is that good and acceptable and perfect will of God." The body can do amazing things, but it's my mind that needs the convincing. If you are just starting this journey of losing weight and getting healthy, start with your mind. Convince yourself that you are worth having a healthy lifestyle. No matter where you start, the Holy Spirit will be right there with you carrying you through the rough patches.

I had a pep talk for myself when I entered the gym telling myself not to leave until I was finished no matter what. So I worked out hard every day; snow days, sleet days, freezing rain days . . . it did not matter what was going on in my life or outside. I am determined not to quit this new lifestyle. Believe it or not, I now look forward to going to the gym. I can't imagine not taking care of the temple that was gifted to me.

Christians should be concerned about losing weight and getting healthy because we are called to go and teach the gospel to all nations. If we are unable to leave our homes due to obesity and illness, how can we be ready for the call to ministry? If we are to follow the example of Christ, then we should really look at how He lived physically. He was very active because His ministry required Him to travel by foot. How are we going to ensure that we spread the good news if we are not well physically, mentally, emotionally, or spiritually? An unhealthy lifestyle is a hindrance to the spreading of the gospel.

Remember, "Greater is he that is in you, than he that is in the world" (1 John 4:4 KJV).

Small Steps to Life Ideas

We are approaching the end of this book and of our twelve-week Losing To Live competition. Hopefully, you have lost weight and have become healthier and stronger. Here are a few last small steps for continuing toward your goal.

What Do You Need to Know about H_2O?

Our blood is made up of 83 percent water. When you do not get enough water, your blood thickens, and when your blood thickens, your body has to work harder to push the blood through your system. This can cause high blood pressure to occur. When I did not drink enough water, I had high blood pressure. Today, I do not have high blood pressure. This is because of a lot of lifestyle changes, and no doubt water was part of that. In the past, I damaged my body through dehydration. So think about it. What kind of damage are you doing to your body because you are not drinking enough water?

Small Food Step

Eat a lot of living food (raw or unprocessed) and limit eating dead food (chemically processed or without nutrients). You want to eat food that is made on a plant, not in a plant. Living food is made by God; it is nutritious and leads to health and life. Dead food is made by man; it is toxic and leads to illness and death.

If you want to live, you have to eat a lot of living food!

Living Food	Dead Food
God	Man
Nutritious	Toxic
Wellness	Illness
Life	Death

Small Exercise Step

Walk 30 minutes at lunchtime on a treadmill. Or better, get out in the sunshine to walk. Walk in place or do simple exercises while waiting for something in your home: water to boil, microwave to beep, during the news, and so on. And stop using power tools outside and go manual—shovel snow, cut grass, rake leaves, and sweep the sidewalks rather than using something with a motor.

Bod4God Victory Guide

Remember that *the victory is in the Victory Guide.* Record your progress on My Progress Report located on page 22.

Week 10: *T* Is for Team: A Group Competition

Bod4God Thought

Christians don't smoke pot, but they do a lot of potlucks.

Bod4God Memory Verse

Two are better than one, because they have a good reward for their labor. (Ecclesiastes 4:9)

Bod4God Reflection/Application Questions

1. Read Ecclesiastes 4:9. What is the value of having a team?

....

....

....

....

....

2. Think of a time when you had to face a struggle on your own, and then compare this to a time when you had a team to help you through a struggle. How was the team helpful to you, and how does this apply to your overall struggle to become healthy?

....

....

....

....

....

3. Read Hebrews 10:24–25 and Ecclesiastes 4:9–12. According to these verses, what is the value of a team?

....

....

....

....

....

4. In what lasting ways has God used the Losing To Live weight-loss challenge to motivate you in becoming a loser?

....

....

....

....

5. Having a lifestyle plan will greatly benefit your health. What changes do you still need to make in the following areas in order to bring about lasting results in your life?

Dedication: Honoring God with My Body

....

....

....

....

Inspiration: Motivating Myself for Change

....

....

....

....

Eat and Exercise: Managing My Habits

....

....

....

....

Team: Building My Circle of Support

....

....

....

....

6. On a scale of 1 to 10, how would you evaluate your health improvements and weight loss since starting this competition? In what ways have you seen your health improve?

....

....

....

....

7. After reading this chapter's Bod4God Close-Up, what can you relate to and what can you take from this person's story to apply to your own life and lifestyle plan?

....

....

....

....

Bod4God Small Steps
to Life Record

What "Skinny Things" Will You Do This Week?

Fill out this chart by indicating: (1) what you will do to eat less to live; (2) what you will do to exercise more to live; and (3) how many average daily ounces of water you will drink. Pick only a few things, and stick with them. Remember that weight loss and maintenance require you to *eat less* and *exercise more*.

Sun.	
Mon.	
Tues.	
Wed.	
Thurs.	
Fri.	
Sat.	

My Bod4God Journal

Teach me, O LORD, the way of Your statutes, and I shall keep
it to the end.

Psalm 119:33

Record what God is telling you to do this week to apply the four keys to
lasting weight loss.

Dedication: Honoring God with My Body

....

....

....

....

Inspiration: Motivating Myself for Change

....

....

....

....

....

Eat and Exercise: Managing My Habits

....

....

....

....

....

Team: Building My Circle of Support

....

....

....

....

....

Frequently Asked Questions

You Can Waste Food or You Can Waist Food

But sanctify the Lord God in your hearts, and always be ready
to give a defense to everyone who asks you a reason for the
hope that is in you, with meekness and fear.

1 Peter 3:15

Question 1

What are your four keys to lasting weight loss?

People ask me, "How did you lose weight?" I tell them, "There are four
keys to weight loss." They are:

1. *Dedication:* For me, weight loss was a matter of bringing together
   my belief system and my behavior. I knew what the Bible taught, yet
   my behavior didn't reflect it. Bringing belief and behavior together
   meant dedicating my body to God and honoring Him with my body.
   My biggest breakthrough was realizing that I needed to depend on
   God to help me. I couldn't do it alone. There's plenty of evidence
   to demonstrate that some people can lose weight and get healthy
   without God, but I'm not one of them. I needed God to help me. I
   had to learn to incorporate walking in the Spirit not just in the pulpit

but also in improving my health. I had to bring those two together in my life.

2. *Inspiration.* To get started and stay on track, you have to find out what motivates you. The fact that you are reading this book is a good start. John 10:10 is the key verse for me in that area. Jesus said, "The thief does not come except to steal, and to kill, and to destroy. I have come that they may have life, and that they may have it more abundantly." The thief, Satan, has an agenda for your life and mine. He comes to steal, kill, and destroy. For many of us, he is using a knife and a fork to do it. Many times, we want to lose weight for some special event. Maybe there's a high school reunion coming up, or a wedding, or some big family event for which you'd like to lose weight. Maybe you do lose weight, but when that event is over, what happens then? Do you gain the weight back? Probably. That's because poor eating habits and lack of movement have become a way of life for you and you still haven't changed your lifestyle. My inspiration is that I want to live the abundant life Jesus promised, and I want it in both quality and quantity.

3. *Eat and Exercise.* I knew I had to manage my habits. I had to learn 1 Thessalonians 4:4, "Each of you should know how to possess his own vessel." "Vessel" here means "body." I had to learn how to possess my body better by improving my habits of eating and exercising—essentially, eating less and exercising more.

4. *Team.* I needed other people to help me in my journey. Proverbs 27:17 says, "As iron sharpens iron, so a man sharpens the countenance of his friend." I had to bring people into my life who could sharpen me when it came to moving toward better health. I had to bring into my life people who knew things I needed to know about health. I had to allow them to impact my life through books, one-on-one encounters, and group-type settings.

Question 2

Can I apply these keys to other addictions in my life?

Yes. These are transferable concepts. In other words, these keys can apply to other areas of your life in which you struggle. With any addiction, whether it is to food, alcohol, nicotine, or any other substance, a physician should be consulted and included in the plan for overcoming it in order to determine the safest course of action for the body.

The Losing To Live message started with a sermon series based on the principle of "losing weight to live better and longer" and showed the ways in which it applies to lots of different areas. We talked about problem areas that have their basis in elevating self above God's Word:

- *Debt* is usually all about self—buying things you can't afford and getting yourself in debt.

- *Anger* is about self. "You offended me. I'm angry with you, and I have a right to be angry."

- *Lust* is about looking at what you want to look at. It's about a strong desire to do what you want to do. It's about acting the way you want to act. You can lust after anything, possessions, people, or pornography, and if it controls your life, you have a problem that needs to be addressed.

- *Stress* has its roots in an attitude that, like an addiction, can control your life and negatively impact it. Stress says, "I can get through life all by myself. I don't need God or anyone else to help me." The same principles apply. In Galatians 2:20, Paul says, "I have been crucified with Christ; it is no longer I who live, but Christ lives in me." It's about dying to self and letting Christ live in and through you.

These principles can be transferred to other areas of your life. As an example, let's use the acrostic D.I.E.T. in dealing with financial debt.

- *Dedication.* Just start out saying, "God, my money belongs to You. You are the owner of it. I'm going to honor You with my money."

- *Inspiration.* Be inspired by reading books about how others have overcome their debt—particularly credit card debt. Dave Ramsey's books on financial freedom are available at all bookstores. Dave had huge debt and had to figure out a way to overcome it. He can inspire you.

- *Eat and Exercise.* Managing your habits. Maybe you have a bad habit of loading up your credit cards with debt. Cut them up. Maybe you have always bought the best of everything—food, clothing, cars. Take another look at your habits and see if you really need top-of-the-line products to accomplish your goals.

- *Team.* Team up with others for whatever problems, stresses, and habits are controlling your life so that you can gain control of them. Form a financial club or an investment club. Work with a team of financial people to learn how to achieve your goals.

Question 3

What does the Bible mean when it says "your body is the temple of the Holy Spirit" (1 Corinthians 6:19)?

First, it means that God's Spirit is a resident in your life. The Scripture indicates that the moment you came to Christ—the moment you were saved—the Holy Spirit came into your life. Jesus said, "I will pray the Father, and He will give you another Helper, that He may abide with you forever—the Spirit of truth, whom the world cannot receive, because it neither sees Him nor knows Him; but you know Him, for He dwells with you and will be in you" (John 14:16–17). God lives in you. Think about it; you as a Christian actually house deity. God doesn't live in a church building. There is nothing sacred about a church building except that it is a place where we come together to corporately worship the Lord. Our bodies are sacred because they are God's temples.

Second, it means that we are to reflect the glory of God. In 1 Corinthians 6:20, Paul says, "For you were bought with a price, therefore glorify God in your body." Because my body is His temple, I should treat it accordingly. In 1 Corinthians 10:31, Paul says, "Therefore, whether you eat or drink or whatever you do, do all to the glory of God." The Bible tells us that one of the ways we can glorify God is through what we eat and what we drink.

Question 4

Does Jesus care whether a person is skinny or fat?

That's an interesting question. I'm not questioning whether Jesus loves us—of course He does. At the same time, He also wants us to be healthy, and that includes not being overweight. He is all about us living. The Bible says He gave His precious blood so that we could live (see John 6:33–35; 1 John 5:11–12).

I have never doubted the love of God in my life. He doesn't love me any more today because I lost weight. But He does care, and He's delighted that I've lost weight. He knows I can live better and probably longer because of my weight loss.

Jesus was nailed to the cross. He suffered and died there because He wanted us to live for all eternity with Him. He also wants us to enjoy our journey here on earth. He cares about our weight problems. He came to give us eternal life in heaven and abundant life on this earth. Being at a proper weight and staying active will give us a better and more abundant life here on earth. So remember that God is not going to love you any less or any more because you lose weight or don't lose weight. It's not about His love, but He does care.

Question 5

Is overeating a sin?

Yes, it is a sin! In 1 Thessalonians 5:23, Paul writes, "Now may the God of peace Himself sanctify you completely; and may your whole spirit, soul, and body be preserved blameless at the coming of our Lord Jesus Christ." God wants to sanctify us wholly—that means our whole spirit and body. Part of being sanctified is having a sanctified eating pattern. So, yes, I think the Bible bears out God's perspective that overeating is a sin.

Question 6

What is your eating and exercise plan?

This is a popular question because people always want to know how I lost weight and how I am keeping it off. There are many ways to lose weight. I've had lots of people try to get me to adopt various plans. They say, "We've got to come see you, and you've got to tell everybody about our plan." That plan may be wonderful. It probably will work for some people, but I'm not about endorsing a single plan. I believe you can lose weight lots of different ways.

The problem isn't that we don't have enough plans. The problem is that we don't stick to the plans or haven't found the right plan for us. My wife and I are not on the same plan. She is losing weight, but she's not losing it the way I am. We are cool with that. She's excited about what she's doing. It's working for her, and I'm proud of her.

What's working for me is a kind of low-carb plan—I guess. I'm eating some carbs but not loading up on them. What I eat is too boring for most people. I'm a boring guy. I don't have to have a big variety of foods in my life to be happy—at least not in this season of life.

A lot of you are different in that way. You've got to come up with all kinds of fresh ideas. You get your cookbooks out and make this and cook that. I'm not that way. Here's what I've begun doing pretty much every day since I embarked on my weight-loss journey:

- *Breakfast:* I start my day by eating old-fashioned oatmeal sweetened with Stevia with raw almonds. It's very nutritious, and I like it a lot. I also eat an apple. With breakfast I drink 16 ounces of water, and I also drink coffee. On my day off, I'll sometimes fix eggs for breakfast.

- *Lunch:* For lunch I get a grilled chicken salad with low-fat dressing. I drink more water. If I go out to eat, that's what I order. A lot of times I'll just go to a grocery store and make a salad from the salad bar. On my day off, I'll make my own salad.

- *Dinner:* For dinner I have lean meat, and five out of seven days a week, that lean meat is chicken. I have green vegetables like broccoli or green beans and water. Many times I'll also have some low-fat and low-sugar yogurt.

- *Snacks:* Planned snacks are important to losing weight. Snacking properly can help keep your metabolism functioning at its peak. I have a late afternoon snack or an early evening snack. This could be a nutritional bar, a piece of fruit, or a few almonds.

When I first started, Friday night was my "cheat night." I funneled all my unhealthy cravings into that one night. If I had been craving ice cream all week, I'd think, *Just two more days until I can go get my ice cream.* But the longer I continue with my small steps to life, the less I need this fix.

I'm on a lifestyle plan, and what that means is that if there is a very special event (I don't try to find a special event every day) like Christmas, I will eat my Christmas meal. I have a good time at the event. I plan to do this the rest of my life. On my plan, you eat Christmas dinner and you enjoy it without guilt. I do try to watch my portion size at the special event. Also, if I know I will be eating a lot at one meal, I cut back at other meals.

Regarding my exercise plan, I started out very slowly. The biggest mistake people make in exercise is to overdo it when they first begin. I slowly built up my routine. Today, I go to a gym and do 35 minutes on the treadmill and 15 different weightlifting activities at least three times a week. My goal is to walk at least 10,000 steps per day. On Sunday nights, I walk the 5K route. It works for me.

Again, you don't have to do what I do. I'm just offering my plan as an idea to get you going. You have to find your own plan.

Question 7

How should I respond when tempted to do unhealthy things?

One of the biggest things to keep you from giving in to temptation is disciplining your mind. What you allow yourself to think about is what you do, and what you do is what you feel. If you want to change your feelings, change your doing. If you want to change your doing, change your thinking.

Every time I gave in to a food temptation, my giving in started with an idea in my mind. I said, "Nice, very nice." And then I ate it. And then I felt bad. So if you want to feel better, you've got to do better. If I'm going to do better, I've got to think better. I have to change my thinking. When I think of that big Hershey's chocolate bar with almonds, I've got to cast down that imagination. I've got to bring every thought into the obedience of Christ (see 2 Corinthians 10:5).

One of the Scripture verses that has helped me a lot is Galatians 6:7–8, "Do not be deceived, God is not mocked; for whatever a man sows, that he will also reap. For he who sows to his flesh will of the flesh reap corruption, but he who sows to the Spirit will of the Spirit reap everlasting life." Do you want corruption or life? I want life. So I think a lot about life, and that begins to change my feelings and my actions.

Question 8

What can I do about overeating because of the stress in my life?

A lot of people eat for comfort. They're under a lot of stress, so they eat. As I told you earlier, many of us who come from the South associate high-fat, rich foods with comfort. It's what we grew up with. It's comforting to us to eat those things.

The Bible calls us to turn to Christ rather than food. Philippians 4:6–7 says, "Be anxious for nothing, but in everything by prayer and supplication, with thanksgiving, let your requests be made known to God; and the peace of God, which surpasses all understanding, will guard your hearts and minds through Christ Jesus." There is a direct correlation between prayer and peace. And that's "peace," not "piece." Make sure you get the spelling right. What can you do about overeating because of the stress in your life? Turn to Christ rather than food.

Question 9

Why does the Bible say that bodily exercise profits little?

First Timothy 4:8 is an interesting verse. We've talked about it before, but I want to highlight it here in a special way. At the time Paul wrote this verse, people had bodily exercise every day. They lived a life that was more intense physically than any gym workout today. As a carpenter, Jesus was a physical worker. In His time, people walked everywhere they went. They had no power tools or electronic conveniences to do the heavy work. Life itself was a workout. When this Scripture verse was read by its original recipients, they would have recognized immediately that it was meant to be a comparison between the physical and the spiritual.

The physical is temporary, so exercise profits the physical body a little. Spiritual exercise lasts forever. It is eternal. We need both physical and spiritual exercise. Growing Christians know that their spiritual exercise is of more eternal value than their physical exercise, yet they need physical exercise to keep the body functioning at peak efficiency.

Question 10

Is it necessary to measure my food?

Men's Health magazine had a small article on writing down what you eat. It said that, "Those who kept a food record for three weeks or longer lost 3.5 pounds more than those who didn't."[1] While most men and many women don't like to write down everything they put in their mouths (I don't write anything down, but I am very mindful about what I eat), keeping a food record appears to work. Even if you only do it for a few weeks, writing down what you eat will help you know how many calories you are actually taking in. Don't forget to write down all those bites you take while cooking or cleaning up after dinner. They all count and add up quickly.

Question 11

How can I know what I'm putting in my mouth?

Nutritional information for food is readily available. Bookstores carry many varieties of calorie counter books and booklets that contain all the nutrient information you need. Many of these books are small enough to carry in your pocket so that you can consult them and make wise choices whenever you're eating at a chain restaurant or fast-food franchise. Also, most major food franchises offer their foods' nutrition information right on the menu as well as online. It is also easy to search for nutritional information on the internet or by using an app on your smartphone. Here's an interesting comparison between the standard cheeseburger and higher-calorie-level offerings as listed on the websites of America's largest fast-food burger restaurants. I hate to even contemplate the fat grams in some of these burgers!

Example: Hamburgers	Calories
McDonald's Cheeseburger®	290
McDonald's Double Quarter Pounder with Cheese®	740
Burger King Cheeseburger®	270
Burger King Triple Whopper®	1,160
Wendy's Jr. Cheeseburger®	280
Wendy's Baconator®	940
Dairy Queen GrillBurger™ with Cheese®	520
Dairy Queen 1/2 lb. FlameThrower® GrillBurger™®	950
Sonic Drive-In Cheeseburger®	750
Sonic Drive-In Bacon Double Cheeseburger®	1,240

A Bod4God Close-Up

It's Never Too Late to Change

John Gandy
Lost 46 pounds

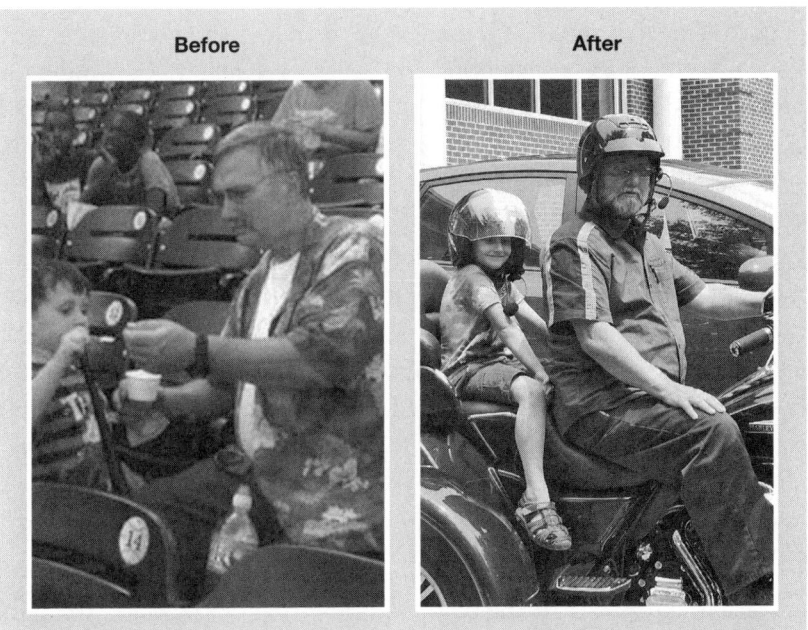

Before   After

Working nights took a toll on my health. I worked three-shift rotations for twenty-five years. When I was younger, I was able to eat whatever and whenever, and my body's metabolism and physical labor were able to keep my weight reasonable. When you do shift work, your sleep and eating patterns are all over the place. One week you eat with your family like a normal person, the next you never see them because you work the 3 p.m.–11 p.m. shift, so you eat whatever you can—chili for breakfast at 2 p.m., spaghetti for dinner at 7 p.m., and your family's leftovers when you get home at midnight. Then you go to bed. The next week is even worse. I used to eat leftovers for breakfast at 10 p.m., a starchy lunch at 4 a.m., and then leftovers again at 8 a.m. before getting into bed. Then the next week you start all over again.

I ignored my weight until my doctor was concerned with my cholesterol levels. He sent me to a nutritionist to help me adjust my eating habits before the cholesterol turned into a serious problem. I also joined a national weight-loss program and lost a lot of weight. However, old habits die hard, and I put the weight back on. At sixty-four years old weighing 239 pounds with high cholesterol, I knew I needed to make a drastic change. I had a family that was counting on me, and I wanted to be around for them for a long time. I knew what to do, I had done it before, and I could do it again. But I didn't.

I started attending the Losing To Live Weight Loss Competition at Capital Baptist Church in Annandale, Virginia. The principles taught by Pastor Steve really hit home, and I found that I had a renewed motivation to change. My inspiration was my family. I wanted to be healthy so that I was around for my family and my youngest son. When I focused on the fact that my body is the temple of God and that He intended for us to take care of that temple so we can be used by Him, things changed. I couldn't serve Him because I was so exhausted and out of breath. I learned that gluttony is just as bad as smoking—it was my sin of choice. Praise God, I have been able to deal with this sin, which has enabled me to lose a total of 46 pounds since joining the program.

I learned in Losing To Live and through my team leader to start taking small steps to life to change the old, unhealthy habits that I had settled into. I started replacing junk food with water and healthier foods, and I was amazed that it didn't take long for the craving for junk food to go away altogether. I was slowly retraining my body to crave healthy and good food. I purchased a pedometer to measure my walking and committed to the goal of 10,000 steps a day. That helped keep me moving. I only wished I had started this process when I was younger. However, I am a testament that it is never too late to change.

I still struggle with skipping meals, especially when I get busy with work and don't have time to eat. Thankfully, I have my Losing To Live team to support me and hold me accountable when I start to struggle. I love that they encourage me, and I can encourage them. You don't have to walk the road of getting healthy alone. Join a team of losers to come alongside you and help. I can go into my team meetings, and if I have gained weight, no one condemns or judges me, and if I have lost weight, everyone celebrates with me. The support is invaluable to the process.

God has given me a seven-year-old son, and I want to watch him grow up and become a man. I want him to have the example of exercise as a child so when he is old, he will already have that habit instilled in his life and not have to work at being fit like I did. I thank and praise God that my cholesterol is no longer a problem. It has been normal for over a year, and my doctor is well pleased. I am thankful that I am able through the Losing To Live program to gain the support I need but also to give support to others who are struggling just like I was. I want to be an example for others, an example of what God can do in you and through you when you dedicate your body to Him. Find an accountability partner to hold you up so that you don't have to take this journey alone. Remember that you didn't get to where you are in one day, so don't expect to lose it all in one week. Look at the long-term view; any movement is better than none. Lastly, if you could do it on your own, you wouldn't be reading this book. Turn it over to God and don't give up. You can do it.

Bod4God Victory Guide

Remember that *the victory is in the Victory Guide*. Record your progress on My Progress Report located on page 22.

Week 11: Frequently Asked Questions

Bod4God Thought

You can waste food or you can waist food.

Bod4God Memory Verse

But sanctify the Lord God in your hearts, and always be ready to give a defense to everyone who asks you a reason for the hope that is in you, with meekness and fear. (1 Peter 3:15)

Bod4God Reflection/Application Questions

Answer the following questions in your own words. How does each question apply to you? Use back-up Scripture when possible.

1. What are the four keys to lasting weight loss?

....

....

....

....

2. How can you apply these keys to other addictions in your life?

....

....

....

....

3. What does the Bible mean when it says "your body is the temple of the Holy Spirit"?

....

....

....

....

....

4. Does Jesus care whether a person is skinny or fat?

....

....

....

....

....

5. Is overeating a sin? Why or why not?

....

....

....

....

....

6. What is your eating and exercise plan?

....

....

....

....

....

7. How should you respond when tempted to do unhealthy things?

....
....
....
....
....

8. What can you do about overeating because of the stress in your life?

....
....
....
....
....

9. Why does the Bible say that bodily exercise profits little?

....
....
....
....
....

10. Is it necessary to measure your food? Why or why not?

....
....
....
....
....

11. How can you know what you are putting in your mouth?

    ....

    ....

    ....

    ....

    ....

12. After reading this chapter's Bod4God Close-Up, what can you relate to and what can you take from this person's story to apply to your own life and lifestyle plan?

    ....

    ....

    ....

    ....

    ....

Bod4God Small Steps
to Life Record

What "Skinny Things" Will You Do This Week?

Fill out this chart by indicating: (1) what you will do to eat less to live; (2) what you will do to exercise more to live; and (3) how many average daily ounces of water you will drink. Pick only a few things, and stick with them. Remember that weight loss and maintenance require you to *eat less* and *exercise more*.

Sun.	
Mon.	
Tues.	
Wed.	
Thurs.	
Fri.	
Sat.	

My Bod4God Journal

Teach me, O Lord, the way of Your statutes, and I shall keep it to the end.

Psalm 119:33

Record what God is telling you to do this week to apply the four keys to lasting weight loss.

Dedication: Honoring God with My Body

....
....
....
....

Inspiration: Motivating Myself for Change

....
....
....
....

Eat and Exercise: Managing My Habits

....
....
....
....

Team: Building My Circle of Support

....

....

....

....

....

Your Bod4God Lifestyle Plan

Nothing Tastes So Good as a Bod4God Feels

It's time to commit! Our conclusion isn't really a conclusion; it's a beginning—the beginning of a new way of life. So how do you get started on this new lifestyle? You do it by making a commitment.

A Scripture to guide you in your commitment is 2 Corinthians 7:1: "Therefore, having these promises, beloved, let us cleanse ourselves from all filthiness of the flesh and spirit, perfecting holiness in the fear of God."

I've done my best to share God's Word with you. You now have the tools you need to get on the Bod4God lifestyle path. It's time for commitment. It's time to cleanse your body from all those things that would keep you from having a Bod4God. It's time to act on what you know is true.

Will you make a commitment to do it? If so, fill out your Bod4God Commitment Form and your Bod4God New Lifestyle Plan. Sign the commitment form, and when times get tough, go back and reread the commitment you made. Follow your new lifestyle plan and continue to build on your small steps to life in order to achieve lasting weight loss. You will never regret it.

My Bod4God Commitment Form

Now that you have read this book and are fully convinced you need to make lifestyle changes, it's time to make a commitment to losing weight and keeping it off.

Dedication: Honoring God with My Body

Walk in the Spirit, and you shall not fulfill the lust of the flesh.

Galatians 5:16

Inspiration: Motivating Myself for Change

The thief does not come except to steal, and to kill, and to destroy. I have come that they may have life, and that they may have it more abundantly.

John 10:10

Eat and Exercise: Managing My Habits

Each of you should know how to possess his own vessel in sanctification and honor.

1 Thessalonians 4:4

Team: Building My Circle of Support

Two are better than one, because they have a good reward for their labor.

Ecclesiastes 4:9

Knowing that my body is made by God and for God, I commit myself to a healthy lifestyle.

Name ....Date ....

My Bod4God New Lifestyle Plan

Take time now to summarize your current lifestyle plan and the small steps to life that you have made so far. Remember, your lifestyle plan continues to be a work in progress, so keep making those small steps to life.

My New Nutritional Plan

How much water will you drink each day? (Remember, a good estimate of how much water to drink is to take your body weight in pounds and divide that number in half. That gives you the number of ounces of water per day that you need to drink.)

....

....

....

What will you eat for breakfast?

....

....

....

....

What will you eat for lunch?

....

....

....

....

....

What will you eat for dinner?

....

....

....

....

....

What will you eat for snacks?

....

....

....

....

....

My New Exercise Plan

What kind of exercise will you do? Fill in your exercise routine in the following chart.

Sun.	
Mon.	
Tues.	

Wed.

Thurs.

Fri.

Sat.

Bod4God Thoughts

For as he thinks in his heart, so is he.

Proverbs 23:7

Your thought life is so important to your success in losing weight. In fact, weight loss begins in your mind with a determination to get started and to stay the course and make the changes necessary to reach your goals, even when it gets tough. In order to help you keep your thought life positive and focused on your goals, I created the following Bod4God thoughts for you to ponder as you go through your twelve-week lifestyle change. I am confident that they will stick with you and will assist you along the way.

Week 1: Your body was made by God and for God.

Week 2: Eat less and exercise more.

Week 3: If food gets near you, it will get in you.

Week 4: The more you move, the more you lose.

Week 5: Short-term pleasure is not worth long-term pain.

Week 6: What you eat in private, you wear in public.

Week 7: Eat for your health, not your happiness.

Week 8:   It is better to exercise an hour a day than to be dead 24 hours a day.

Week 9:   Don't try to lose weight alone; join a team of losers.

Week 10:   Christians don't smoke pot, but they do a lot of potlucks.

Week 11:   You can waste food or you can waist food.

Week 12:   Nothing tastes so good as a Bod4God feels.

Bod4God Memory Verses

Then Jesus said to those Jews who believed Him, "If you abide in My word, you are My disciples indeed. And you shall know the truth, and the truth shall make you free."

John 8:31–32

The Bible is the absolute truth. Jesus said that by knowing the truth we can be set free from sin. Understand that the battle of the bulge will be won or lost in the mind; therefore, fill your mind with the Word of God.

There are eleven memory verses for you to learn throughout the program. Memorize one verse each week if possible. These verses will encourage you to stay true to your goal of a better Bod4God. Write one verse on a card each week and post the card in your car, on your bathroom mirror, on your computer screen, or wherever you'll see it first thing in the morning.

Week 1: Colossians 1:16

For by Him all things were created that are in heaven and that are on earth, visible and invisible, whether thrones or dominions or principalities or powers. All things were created through Him and for Him.

Week 2: Matthew 16:24–25

Then Jesus said to his disciples, "If anyone desires to come after Me, let him deny himself, and take up his cross, and follow Me. For whoever desires to save his life will lose it, but whoever loses his life for My sake will find it."

Week 3: Galatians 5:16

Walk in the Spirit, and you shall not fulfill the lust of the flesh.

Week 4: Romans 10:9

If you confess with your mouth the Lord Jesus and believe in your heart that God has raised Him from the dead, you will be saved.

Week 5: John 10:10

The thief does not come except to steal, and to kill, and to destroy. I have come that they may have life, and that they may have it more abundantly.

Week 6: Philippians 4:13

I can do all things through Christ who strengthens me.

Week 7: 1 Thessalonians 4:4

Each of you should know how to possess his own vessel in sanctification and honor.

Week 8: 1 Corinthians 10:31

Therefore, whether you eat or drink, or whatever you do, do all to the glory of God.

Week 9: Psalm 51:12

Restore to me the joy of Your salvation, and uphold me by Your generous Spirit.

Week 10: Ecclesiastes 4:9

Two are better than one, because they have a good reward for their labor.

Week 11: 1 Peter 3:15

But sanctify the Lord God in your hearts, and always be ready to give a defense to everyone who asks you a reason for the hope that is in you, with meekness and fear.

How Other Churches Are Using the Bod4God Program

My great passion is to see this program spread to churches everywhere. And it has begun. Here are a few inspiring stories.

Michael Parks

Woodstream Church
Mitchellville, Maryland

After hearing Pastor Steve Reynolds speak at a men's conference about Losing To Live, I knew that I had to bring it to my church. I am so thankful that Pastor Robert of Woodstream Church embraced the idea as well and supported me in launching the program and making it successful. It has truly transformed the health of our church.

We see it as our duty to teach Christians to take care of themselves in order to better serve God. The Bible says that our lifestyle is a testimony to others, and our lives should glorify God. Jesus was fit, and we are His body. Therefore, we need to pattern ourselves after our Head, our Leader. We must take care of the temples that God has given us.

Our Losing To Live program is such an important ministry in the church because people need to know that they can turn to God to get healthy. It helps people develop a closer relationship with God and take care of their bodies. It has also helped us become a walking testimony of what God can do when you trust Him with all things, including eating. It is so encouraging to see people getting off diabetes and blood pressure medications, and people with knee problems now running marathons.

Pastor Bob teaches us through his preaching about the importance of health, and he also models fitness and health in his own life. His positive example is a huge factor in the success of our program. He also supports us by allowing weekly announcements in the church bulletin, poster boards, and a registration table for signing up for the program and various events, such as different 5K events for our participants to compete in.

The Losing To Live program is life-changing and has helped our church lose over 1,700 pounds. We run our competitions every spring and fall. We use *Bod4God* as our guide. It helps us learn what the Bible says about honoring God with our bodies and taking small steps to life. We also focus on doing fun activities together. Beginning in the spring, a group of members meets after church and bikes the trails of Washington, DC, Maryland, and Virginia. We pray before we start riding, support each other, and have fun fellowshiping along the ride.

Our congregation is very receptive and glad that they can turn to the church for help with weight loss, and they are slowly spreading the message by word of mouth to the community. I want to encourage you to get your church focused on health. Make sure that the people in your church understand that this is a commitment to a lifestyle that is God-honoring and not self-gratifying.

Sue Ryno

Monclova Road Baptist Church
Monclova, Ohio

I first heard of Steve Reynolds and Losing To Live through the ministry of First Place 4 Health and their newsletters. I would read Pastor Steve's articles, and then one day I saw his book *Bod4God: Twelve Weeks to Lasting Weight Loss* in the LifeWay Christian Store. It was as if God was speaking to me on this issue of health and wellness. I was shocked when I first learned that two-thirds of Americans are considered obese or overweight. I believe that this problem can be a result of an empty spiritual dimension, making food a god to fill up the emptiness and loneliness that only God can fill.

The church today can have a part in overcoming this epidemic by showing people that God is the answer for their problems, not food. We are not our own, but rather we are bought with a price. Our bodies are a temple, and we cannot be a good witness for Christ if we are displaying our bellies as our god. This is why we started offering the Losing To Live Weight Loss Competition at our church.

We have offered three competitions and plan to continue with this ministry. These competitions, which were paired with preaching by Pastor Russ Merrin on the body of the believer being the temple of God and indwelled by the Holy Spirit, have really made a difference in the lives of the people in our church. We have lost over 1,000 pounds! Also, our church events that involve food have offered healthier food choices.

We are so proud of our team members who have achieved great success through the program. Ed, our biggest loser to date, lost 77 pounds, and for the first time, he has put God at the head of his weight-loss goals. Shirley, age seventy-one, lost 21 pounds. Sharon, age sixty-seven, lost 17 pounds and is now off insulin. Madison and Betty suffered from blood pressure and sugar problems but now are doing very well. Another competitor, Donna, was looking for inspiration and found it in this program. She lost 38 pounds and four dress sizes. The program has been so successful and well received in the community that we have even attracted the attention of the media.

Launch the Losing To Live Weight Loss Competition in your church. Follow the *Bod4God* book, be spirited, and ask for helpers. We are excited about the program because weight loss and discipline are tied to the spiritual. Many of our participants have stated that this is the first weight-loss program they completed that incorporated God and His Word. Get started today. You won't be disappointed.

Cheryl Zorko

Westgate Chapel
Edmonds, Washington

I first heard about *Bod4God* and Losing To Live from my brother, Don Ross, a pastor of a church near my own church. I work as an administrative assistant at my home church. My brother was hosting a Losing To Live Weight Loss Competition, and I committed to attend. I faithfully attended the weight-loss group and lost my first 25 pounds. I became so excited about the program that I brought it back to my church, and my pastor embraced the idea of offering the program as a small group and allowing me to lead it. A burden was growing in me to establish a health and wellness ministry at my church so that we can teach people to bring glory to God in all areas of their lives including the physical.

One of the things that I love most about the program is that it really opens our eyes to the truth that gluttony is a sin. It also focuses on losing weight through a team approach and for the right reason. Losing weight with other people in order to honor the Lord is the key. Many members of our groups have been enlightened about making permanent lifestyle changes rather than just finishing a twelve-week diet program. Most people come to that "aha" moment when they realize that this is all about loving the Lord with all that you are. It almost brings tears to my eyes to see the lightbulb come on for so many people involved in the small group around the third or fourth week of the study. We have found the Bod4God videos to be very helpful for great information and inspiration.

I am so thankful that I have been able to lose 58 pounds and have kept it off for almost two years now. I was in love with chocolate and lots of other foods that were horrible for me. I also did not like to exercise, but I now know how important it is, and I see the good results in doing it. Our church has lost approximately 500 pounds since starting our Bod4God small groups. We hold the class three times a year during our fall, winter, and summer terms. We also occasionally offer exercise groups to supplement the program.

Bod4God has truly transformed my life and the lives of many others in our church. My total mind-set about eating has been turned upside down. It's not about me anymore but rather about God and honoring Him. I don't want to sin against Him in any way, shape, or form. My selfishness was sinful, and I have been set free from all of the past and now look to a life of losing to live and bringing glory to the name of Jesus. He is my healer, motivator, strength, and coach. I feel honored to be able to help others achieve what I have through this ministry.

Joseph Tubb

Venture Church
Hattiesburg, Mississippi

Pastor Jeff Clark and his team at Venture Church know that they have their work cut out for them, not just in reaching a community for Christ but also in changing a culture of obesity that plagues our state. Mississippi is the most obese state in the nation; however, Pastor Clark and others like myself in the church have taken on the challenge of turning the tide on the obesity epidemic. After hearing about the Losing To Live program from another pastor in Arkansas, we became determined to start the program at our church.

At Venture Church, we believe that a healthy body promotes a healthy mind, and a healthy mind is ready to learn, worship, and be more open to fulfilling God's plan. Isn't that the goal of what we want for the people in our churches, to be able to see God's plan for their lives and do it? If the fact that Christians are the most overweight people in America isn't enough cause for concern for the church today, we should all look to the Bible for reasons why we should be concerned. God does not want His people to be overweight and out of shape. He does not want His church to be unhealthy and sick, physically or spiritually. God wants His people to be healthy so that they can honor Him and be ready to fulfill the work that He has for them. Healthy Christians can serve more in the church and do more in the world.

We began our health and wellness vision at Venture Church with a sermon series that Pastor Jeff preached entitled "FIT." He talked about why we should be concerned with being good managers of our bodies. It was through this series that our vision was born. We are now educating our church on healthy living through Bod4God growth groups.

We have a big job to do in Mississippi due to our state being so obese and unhealthy. Because the problem in Mississippi is so great, we knew that we could not do it alone. We shared the vision of having churches lead the charge in health and wellness. Praise God, other churches have begun the program. Our goal is to spread the word throughout our entire state so that no matter where a person lives, they can attend a Losing To Live program in a church near them.

We hope that our vision and story encourage you to get started and get started now! Gather teams of people who want to lose weight, get healthy, and dedicate their bodies to God. Thank you, Pastor Steve, for writing a book that not only shows why we should want to live healthier but also shows us how to do it. With a lot of hard work we can hopefully turn the tide of the obesity epidemic not only in Mississippi but in every state.

How to Set Up Your Group Competition

Can people lose weight without a group competition? Yes, they can, but most people do much better when they are part of a community environment. Getting healthy with a larger group provides support that goes a long way in lasting weight loss. We all need connection and a place to share our successes and failures. So don't try to lose weight alone and don't ask your church to either—create teams of losers!

Here is a simple guide for setting up a Losing To Live Weight Loss Competition.

What to Do before the Competition

Step 1: Know Your Purposes

If you are clear about your purposes and can articulate them to your pastor, key leaders, and congregation, you will quickly gain their approval. Christians are the most overweight people group in America, and Losing To Live has been designed to confront and help solve this problem. This biblical program will show people in your church how to lose weight and keep it off through a Bod4God lifestyle. The goal is to change lives one pound at a time.

Step 2: Seek Approval from the Leadership of Your Church

- If you are the *pastor*, inform your key leaders about what you are planning to do and why you are doing it.
- If you are *not the pastor*, go first to your pastor and share your passion to help church members lose weight. Then let the pastor inform the key leaders.

Step 3: Establish Your Schedule and Location

Any time of year is a good time to start a Losing To Live competition because overweight people think about their weight struggle almost every day. The competition takes twelve weeks. Participants meet once a week for 90 minutes. During the first 30 minutes, everyone gets an update on the total weight loss results and watches a Bod4God video. During the remaining hour, participants break into teams for discussion. You will need:

- A place large enough for all participants to meet together and equipped to play the Bod4God videos.
- Smaller rooms or areas where individual teams can meet.
- A private place to put your scale for weigh-ins.

Step 4: Recruit and Assign Leaders

You'll want to recruit a director, team captains, and administrative support to do the weigh-ins and other activities during the sessions. Pray earnestly about who these people should be, as they will be crucial to the success of the program.

Step 5: Organize Your Registration Process

All participants must fill out a Losing To Live Registration Form. The form is part of the Bod4God Video Series Kit which can be found at www. bod4god.org. This form will help you in ordering your participant kits, organizing your teams, and communicating with your participants.

Step 6: Implement Your Promotion Strategy

Your promotion should target your church and your community. A promotional video and other materials are available in the Bod4God Video Series Kit, which can be obtained at www.bod4god.org.

Step 7: Host an Orientation Meeting

Two to three weeks before the first competition, host an orientation meeting for potential participants. The goal of the meeting is to explain how the competition works and then register participants for the upcoming twelve-week competition. Distribute the Losing To Live Fact Sheet and show the orientation video presentation by Pastor Steve Reynolds, both of which are part of the Bod4God Video Series Kit and can be found at www.bod4god.org.

Step 8: Order Your Participant Kits

Each participant should receive an official Losing To Live Participant Kit (available at www.bod4god.org). One person can order the kits for everyone, or each person can order their own kit. The kit contains a copy of the *Bod4God* book by Pastor Steve Reynolds (each participant will need a book to do the Victory Guide exercises that are crucial to success in the program), an official Losing To Live T-shirt, and a refrigerator magnet.

Step 9: Determine Your Teams

After each participant has been registered, divide the enrollees into teams of six to twelve people. Each team should be balanced out between those who need to lose a lot of weight and those who need to lose less weight. Don't worry if you only have one or two teams the first time. As these first teams have success, others will notice and join the program.

Step 10: Set Up Your Weigh-In Procedure

You will need a good-quality scale and a private place for weigh-ins. Have participants come in one at a time to weigh in. For the convenience of participants, the best time to schedule weigh-ins is before and after the meetings. The competition is based on the percentage of weight loss, not the number of pounds lost. Most groups use a Microsoft Excel spreadsheet to do their calculations.

Step 11: Set Up How You Will Communicate with Participants

Get email addresses and phone numbers from all participants. For the best success, the director and the group leaders need to be in contact with the participants on a weekly basis. A little encouragement will go a long way toward helping the participants stay on track.

What to Do During the Competition

Step 1: Conduct Weekly Weigh-Ins

Record the participants' weights each week without comment. Whether they have lost or gained, this is their story to tell. Say nothing to the participant or to anyone else.

Step 2: Conduct Weekly Rally Time

At the rally, announce the total weight loss, individual teams' total weight loss, and some of the top individual losers. Show the Bod4God video that goes with the weekly chapter in the *Bod4God* book (the video series kit is available at www.bod4god.org).

Step 3: Conduct Weekly Small Groups

Most participants will connect best with the program in their small group teams. Each team should choose a team name based on a fruit or vegetable as a rallying cry. During each team meeting, the participants should:

- Go over the information in *Bod4God* chapter by chapter.
- Specifically discuss the weekly Victory Guide assignments, including their "small steps to life."
- Share ideas on what is working for each person.
- Cheer each other's successes.
- Pray together.

Step 4: Conduct a Victory Celebration

Although the weekly rally time is a kind of celebration, you will also want to have a big, final celebratory event. Note that:

- During this last-week celebration, you will change the order of the meeting by having the small group time first and the rally time second. (The small groups will meet first to go over the material in week 12.)
- You will announce the overall weight loss for the entire group and the various teams during the celebration and recognize the individual biggest loser(s).
- You will give each participant a certificate of participation (available in the Bod4God Video Series Kit).
- You should decide if you would like to give out prizes.
- Any food provided for this event should be healthy.
- If you have individuals who have had unusual success, you may want to call in the media to do a story.
- You should rejoice over what God has helped you accomplish together and make sure everyone leaves feeling like a winner.

For more information or to get a complete Losing To Live Weight Loss Competition Group Starter Kit, which includes the *Bod4God* book, Bod-4God Video Series, the official Losing To Live T-shirt, and a refrigerator magnet, visit:

www.bod4god.org

or contact:
Losing To Live
P.O. Box 300
Merrifield, VA 22116
703-635-7100 • 866-596-6008

You may also contact Pastor Steve Reynolds about speaking to your church or organization.

Notes

Week 1 The Anti-Fat Pastor

1. Amy Patterson Neubert, "Study Finds Some Faithful Less Likely to Pass the Plate," *Purdue University News*, August 24, 2006, http://www.purdue.edu/uns/html4ever/2006/06 0824.Ferraro.obesity.html.

2. Mayo Clinic, "Water: How Much Should You Drink Every Day?," September 5, 2014, http://www.mayoclinic.org/healthy-lifestyle/nutrition-and-healthy-eating/in-depth/water/art -20044256?pg=1.

3. These are general guidelines for water consumption. However, there are certain circumstances when an individual may be on medications or have underlying kidney disease or other chronic illness in which too much water is detrimental to health. As with any general health guidelines, please consult with your personal physician or health care provider for specific recommendations based upon your medication profile, health history, and level of exercise.

Week 3 *D* Is for Dedication

1. "Being Overweight Is Not Good," ChristiaNet, http://christiannews.christianet.com /1190131185.htm.

2. Krista M. C. Cline and Kenneth F. Ferraro, "Does Religion Increase the Prevalence and Incidence of Obesity in Adulthood?," *Journal for the Scientific Study of Religion* 45, no. 2 (2006): 269–81, http://www.ncbi.nlm.nih.gov/pmc/articles/PMC3358928/.

3. Neubert, "Study Finds Some Faithful Less Likely to Pass the Plate."

4. Ibid.

5. Frank M. Sacks et al., "Comparison of Weight-Loss Diets with Different Compositions of Fat, Protein, and Carbohydrates," *New England Journal of Medicine* 360, no. 9 (2009): 859–73, doi:10.1056/NEJMoa0804748.

6. Lawrence J. Appel et al., "Comparative Effectiveness of Weight-Loss Interventions in Clinical Practice," *New England Journal of Medicine* 365, no. 21 (2011): 1959–68, doi:10.1056 /NEJMoa1108660.

7. Ibid.

8. M. L. Dansinger et al., "Comparison of the Atkins, Ornish, Weight Watchers, and Zone Diets for Weight Loss and Heart Disease Risk Reduction: A Randomized Trial," *Journal of the American Medical Association* 293, no. 1 (2005): 43–53.

Week 4 *D* Is for More Dedication

1. *The Free Dictionary*, s.v. "discipline," http://www.thefreedictionary.com/discipline.

Week 5 *I* Is for Inspiration

1. Don Jeffries, "Pastor, Father, Addict," *Reader's Digest* (Canadian), June 1992, 201.

Week 7 *E* Is for Eat

1. Emily Callahan, personal correspondence with the author, August 15, 2011. Used by permission.
2. Dr. Baroni, personal correspondence with the author, April 13, 2015. Used by permission.

Week 8 *E* Is for Exercise

1. Lin Yang and Graham A. Colditz, "Prevalence of Overweight and Obesity in the United States, 2007–2012," *JAMA Internal Medicine* 175, no. 8 (2015):1412–13.
2. US Department of Health & Human Services, "Active Living," May 2014, http://www.surgeongeneral.gov/priorities/prevention/strategy/active-living.html.
3. Jeannie Blocher, personal correspondence with the author, July 7, 2015. Used by permission.

Week 9 *T* Is for Team: A Personal Challenge

1. National Institutes of Health, "Overweight and Obesity Statistics," updated October 2012, http://www.niddk.nih.gov/health-information/health-statistics/Pages/overweight-obesity-statistics.aspx.
2. "Adult Obesity in the United States," The State of Obesity, September 2014. http://stateofobesity.org/adult-obesity/.
3. National Institutes of Health, "Clinical Guidelines on the Identification, Evaluation, and Treatment of Overweight and Obesity in Adults," September 1998, http://www.nhlbi.nih.gov/guidelines/obesity/ob_gdlns.pdf.
4. Mayo Clinic, "Weight Loss: Strategies for Success," February 26, 2014, http://www.mayoclinic.org/healthy-lifestyle/weight-loss/in-depth/weight-loss/art-20047752.

Week 10 *T* Is for Team: A Group Competition

1. Becky Stephenson, personal correspondence with the author, April 14, 2015. Used by permission.

Week 11 Frequently Asked Questions

1. Maria Masters, ed., "Weight-Loss Bulletin: Write Off the Pounds," *Men's Health*, February 2009, 38.

Steve Reynolds, America's "Anti-Fat Pastor," has served as the senior pastor of Capital Baptist Church in suburban Washington, DC, since 1982. He is the creator of the Losing To Live Weight Loss Competition. His story of dramatic weight loss has been featured on local, national, and international media, including *The View*. Steve is a graduate of Liberty University and Theological Seminary. Learn more at www.bod4god.org.

Be the First to Hear about Other New Books from REVELL!

Sign up for announcements about new and upcoming titles at

RevellBooks.com/SignUp

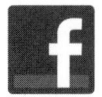

Don't miss out on our great reads!

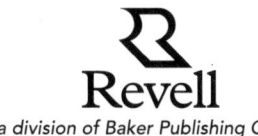

Revell

a division of Baker Publishing Group

www.RevellBooks.com